Parting
the
Curtains

Parting *the* Curtains

A Woman's Handbook of Sex and Sexuality

Ditza Katz, PT, PhD &
Ross Lynn Tabisel, LCSW, PhD

Katz-Tabi Publications

Women's Therapy Center
54 Sunnyside Blvd., Suite A
Plainview, NY 11803
516.576.1118
www.womentc.com

Cover and book design by Ryan Scheife www.mayflydesign.com
Illustrations by Anne C. Reiner
Cover images © Shutterstock.com

The information provided in this book is meant for educational purposes only and
should not take the place of prompt medical care.

Printed in USA
ISBN 978-0-9700298-6-7
Kindle edition: 978-0-9700298-7-4
e-Pub edition: 978-0-9700298-8-1

Also by these authors:
Private Pain: It's About Life, Not Just Sex
Understanding Vaginismus & Dyspareunia
ISBN 978-0-9700298-3-6, Third Edition
Kindle edition: 978-0-9700298-5-0
e-Pub edition: 978-0-9700298-4-3

To Syvonne, Liat, and Hannah, with much love.

To my Mom, Shula (Zita):

Your dream of becoming a physician was shattered when deported to the
Auschwitz-Birkenau extermination camp where you lost your youth and
identity and became prisoner #A15975, a number that was tattooed
onto your left forearm as an eternal reminder.

You were tortured by the Nazi machine. You lost your parents, siblings, and most
of your loved ones. You were hungry, cold, and scared. You witnessed unimaginable
atrocities. You survived. You rebuilt. You dreamt. You lost a love. You endured a
detention camp en route to Israel. You had a family. You developed a successful
career as a fashion designer. You lived despite always fighting from within.
And through it all, you nurtured within you the power and ability to be
the best mother one could ask for. I will never come close
to understanding how.

This book is dedicated to you for giving me life, love, and eternal inspiration.

In just a few years the last living witness to the Holocaust will be gone.

WE MUST NEVER FORGET!

—DITZA

My dedication goes to the women who have played such an important role in my life:

- Grandma Sis, who always praised me and taught me to speak my mind.

- Aunt Gloria, who made me feel like I was her daughter.
- Aunt Peggy, who taught me that friendship is
something that should be valued, forever.

- My mother-in-law Hilda, who was always there to listen.

- Shula (Savta), whose strength and perseverance
showed me that one can always forge forward.

- Shelly, my sister, who in her last days asked me to take care of our brother
and to always be there for Madison & Mason. I will never stop filling her
final request.

- My daughter Sloane, who believes so strongly
in everything I do, and who will carry on my work.

A special tribute to my mother, "Dukie." Had she still been here, she would have been
carrying around this book and showing it off to everyone she knew. Mom, you always
believed in me, were proud of me, and thought I could do anything. You gave me the
ability to see the world as good, to care, to be kind to others, and to make
lemonade out of lemons! I will forever love you "to the moon and back again."

Also, with much love, to the men in my life who believe in me and my work:

- My brother Russell, who gets red every time
he tells someone what I do, yet is so proud!

- My brother Steven, who took care of our Mom & Dad.
I truly understand what this meant; Thank you!

- My Dad, whose last words to me were,
"I love you, you make me proud." I know you are glowing.

- My son Brett, who is unconditionally proud of me.

Last but not least, to my husband Lenny, who puts up with my coming home late from
work, and with waking up at night to take phone calls, and who - in his quiet ways - is
always there.

—ROSS

Acknowledgments

We thank our patients for permitting us to enter their innermost personal space at time of pain and distress, for sharing with us their fears and worries, and for entrusting us with guiding them through the biased, complex maze of female sex and sexuality.

A special Thank You to Brett Tabisel for brilliantly parting the curtains.

Our deepest thanks to our editor, Sara Sherbill, who helped translate our ideas into readable prose, and whose passion for women's health added a great deal to our project.

Special appreciation to the following individuals who devoted time and energy to reading the manuscript and giving us their thoughtful input: Naomi Bodek, Ilene Drapkin, Rachel Miner, Megan Walker, and Staci Wasserberger.

We are also grateful to our own life experiences that made us understand female sex and sexuality from within.

Table of Contents

CHAPTER FOUR

CHAPTER FIVE

CHAPTER SIX

Introduction

This book is the product of over two decades of listening to and treating women in our New York clinic, where we have guided our patients through a range of sexual challenges—everything from the inability to have intercourse to how to have an orgasm to contraceptive counseling. Initially, we relied on our blog to share the questions and concerns we encountered most frequently. While we still love our blog - and update it frequently! - over time, it became clear to us that the anecdotes and experiences we'd been collecting should be turned into an accessible, handbook addressing the real-life issues that so many women face. Whether you use this book as a reference, an educational tool, or a preventative manual, our aim is that it will answer your questions in a way that embraces female sexuality without medicalizing or sensationalizing it.

In a sense, one could say that we began writing this book when we opened the doors to The Women's Therapy Center in 1996. As readers will discover, our clinical approach is based on the underlying premise that knowledge is power, and that the more women know about how their bodies work, the better equipped they will be to explore their sexuality, and to deal with dilemmas when they arise. We are also believers in the inextricable link between body and mind, and in addressing women's physical and emotional needs as a whole, in a coordinated, holistic manner. Thankfully, there is growing awareness in the medical community that our emotions play a vital role in our health, and vice versa. In our practice, we try to illuminate this connection, helping women to understand that what goes on in the bedroom is largely influenced by what's going on in a woman's mind. Last but not least, we believe that sexuality is a gift—something to be enjoyed and celebrated—at all stages of a woman's life, regardless of her age, religion, sexual orientation, or relationship status.

In writing this book we wanted to create a practical, goal-oriented guide grounded in our clinical experience—for women young or old, straight or gay, partnered or single. While all names and identifying details have been changed to protect our patients' privacy, our objective in these pages is to let the voices and experiences of real women shine through, and remind other women that they are not alone. From fertility and menopause, to emotional health and relationships, to urogynecological restoration and post-cancer rehabilitation, we have tried to put together a reader-friendly reference that can help each and every woman navigate her sexual journey armed with up-to-date information and a good dose of self-respect. Every effort was made to use gender-inclusive language wherever possible. However, in some instances we have relied on the use of a single pronoun for the sake of clarity.

Our intention is that this book will also be used by mental health and medical professionals, as well as by members of the clergy, who find themselves counseling individuals and couples grappling with sexual difficulties. Although recent years have brought an increased awareness of women's health, there are still plenty of misconceptions out there; this book represents our contribution to clarifying some of them.

To you, our readers—we hope that this book will inspire you to advocate for yourself and to seek solutions. We also hope it will begin a dialogue for you—with yourself, your friends, or your partner.

There is much more to the topic of female sex and sexuality but, for the sake of practicality, the content was limited and was not meant to be comprehensive. For further discussion, visit our website at womentc.com, and email us with your input or questions.

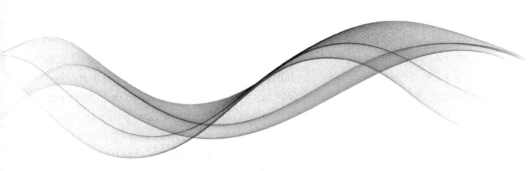

Chapter One

Getting to Know Your Body

The Basics

Do I look normal down there? This question is among those we hear most often. After all, most of us haven't seen too many other vulvas (unlike the penis, which is visible to the naked eye), so it's hard to have a sense of what we're "supposed to" look like. But the truth is that there's no "supposed to" because, as with other body parts, no two vulvas are exactly the same.

For many years now, showing women their genitals has been a mandatory component of our patient care. The following are some of the comments we've heard as our patients look at their vulvas for the first time, and when shown their vaginas through an open speculum:

▶ I cannot do it . . .
▶ I am very ugly down there
▶ Do I look normal?
▶ I am going to throw up
▶ It does not look right
▶ I was told to never touch or look there

▶ Wow, is that it?
▶ How cool!
▶ I can finally stop worrying about it . . .
▶ Where is my hymen?
▶ I was never able to do that before!

1

As some of the comments above illustrate, women are often concerned about the shape, size, and color of their genitals. Some are particularly worried about their inner lips - the labia minora - and why one is bigger/smaller/longer/shorter than the other. The answer is quite simple: to each her own. In some women, the inner lips rest within the outer lips, while in others they may protrude, making them visible even when the outer lips aren't separated. For others, their inner lips may be so small that it may be difficult to find them at all. And for some, an inner lip may be missing altogether. None of these variations will affect a woman's ability to experience sexual pleasure, nor should they be cause for embarrassment or concern.

When it comes to color, some express alarm that their vulva is "too red," "too dark," or "too light." The fact is that the natural color of the vulva may undergo changes in response to hormonal shifts, sexual activity, certain dermatologic conditions, age, even levels of hydration. So unless you have other symptoms that warrant medical attention, there is nothing to worry about.

Many of us have been raised to regard our vaginas as though they're invisible: not to be looked at, touched, or discussed. Unlike boys, who encounter their penises at an early age, and, through the act of urination, are instructed to touch them, many girls are simply not taught about their own genitals, let alone encouraged to explore them. The result is that even as grown women, we're not always sure where things are and how they work.

One of the primary goals of our practice is to change that reality—one woman at a time. So read on, and take the brave step of getting to know your own body.

Meet Your Vulva and Vagina

Here's an overview of the vulva and the vagina, followed by an exercise you can try on your own.

Outer lips (or labia majora): The external folds of skin, one on each side, which typically have the same "puffy" look in most women, and which act as a cushion against the male pubic bone during intercourse.

Female genitals

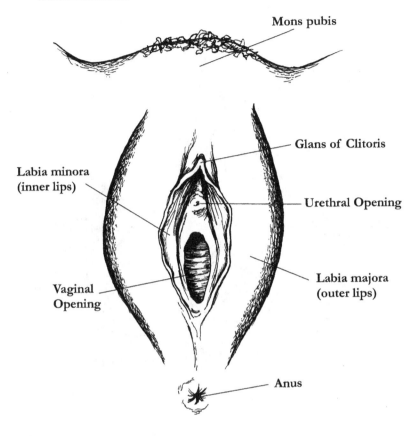

Mons pubis

Glans of Clitoris

Labia minora
(inner lips)

Urethral Opening

Labia majora
(outer lips)

Vaginal
Opening

Anus

Vulva: The external genital organs; it is everything you see when you part the outer lips.

Inner lips (or labia minora): The internal skin folds that are visible once the outer lips are parted. The size of the inner lips varies greatly among women.

Vestibule: the area within the inner lips that includes the vaginal and urethral openings.

Urethral opening (urinary meatus): This is the visible end of the urethra through which we release urine out of the body. The urethral opening is located just above the vaginal opening within the vestibule,

The Clitoris

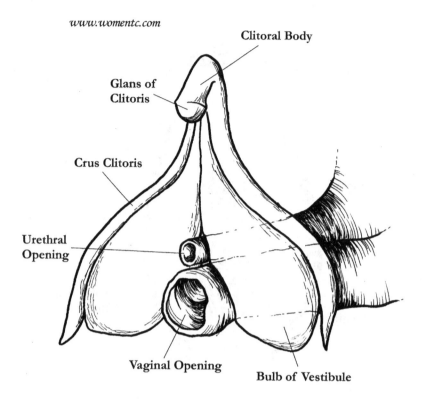

Clitoral Body

Glans of Clitoris

Crus Clitoris

Urethral Opening

Vaginal Opening

Bulb of Vestibule

and is surrounded by protective fatty, estrogenic-rich tissue, which gives it the appearance of a small, soft blob of tissue. Continuing inward from the urethral opening is the itself, which terminates at the bladder. The urethra lies parallel to the lower third of the vagina, as if it were a pipe that runs along its ceiling, thus making it intimately connected to vaginal sensations. The underside of the urethra, which forms the ceiling of the vagina, is also lined with fatty, estrogenic tissue, which serves as a cushion during vaginal penetrations of any kind (tampons, intercourse, etc.). When estrogen is compromised, however, as in the case of menopause, the protective estrogenic tissue begins to thin-out, making the urethra more reactive to penetration.

Vaginal opening (introitus): Found within the inner lips, at the very bottom of the genital oval. It is the entrance to the vaginal canal, which continues into the pelvis and ends at the cervix.

Cervix: A donut-shaped structure with a small opening at the center, which serves as the entrance to the uterus (womb).

Clitoris: A woman's primary erogenous organ, similar in size and feel to a (very sensitive!) small pebble. We can only see its tip—glans clitoris—which is situated above the urethral and vaginal openings. In other words, *the clitoris is not inside the vagina*, a common misconception. The clitoris is shaped like a wishbone with its "legs" (right crus + left crus = crura) extending down on either side of the vagina and containing spongy tissue (corpus cavernosum) that engorges with blood upon arousal, similar to penile erection. The skin fold covering the glans clitoris—clitoral hood, or prepuce—is the female's analog to the male's foreskin.

Women need clitoral stimulation for sexual arousal, whether by direct contact—with a hand, tongue, or vibrator, for example—or indirect contact, when the shaft of the penis rubs the clitoris and/or tugs on the inner lips just the right way during intercourse, leading to what is known as a "**vaginal orgasm**" (a subject we discuss in greater length in Chapter Five).

What About the Hymen?

Although there remains a stubborn misconception that a "virgin" will always have an intact hymen, the truth is that most women age 20 and older do not have a hymen, or only have a partial hymen, even if they have never had any vaginal penetration. How is this possible, you ask? Because unlike the prepubescent and adolescent vagina, the adult vaginal tissue has been under the influence of estrogen for several years, which causes it to elasticize and expand.

That said, there is no shortage of myths floating around about the hymen, so let's dispel the two most common right away:

▶ You cannot break a hymen by exercising, bike riding, or riding a horse
▶ The hymen is not visible through the genital lips; its presence can only be confirmed with an internal examination

---

Explore

Just like we encourage our patients, we encourage you, too, to look at your genitals and get to know them a bit better. Using a mirror, explore the outer lips (labia majora), inner lips (labia minora), clitoris, and clitoral hood, as well as the place where your urine comes out (urethral meatus), and the vaginal opening located right below it. Don't be surprised if the vagina seems closed up—this is quite normal, especially for women who have not had multiple vaginal births.

If you can, insert a lubricated finger into your vagina up to your middle knuckle, and gently move your finger around to get a sense of what your vagina feels like. With your finger still inside, try squeezing your muscles as though to prevent yourself from passing urine or from making a bowel movement. If you are able to feel your pelvic floor muscles tightening, you have just done a Kegel exercise by contracting your PC (pubococcygeus) muscle. While your finger is inside your vagina, you may want to feel around: above is the underside of your pubic bone and the urethra that is just under it; below is the rectal canal; the sides feel soft and flexible like the inside of your mouth.

Kegel Exercises

Kegel exercises are the squeezing of the muscles of the pelvic floor, named after Dr. Arnold Kegel (1894-1981), a gynecologist who pioneered this approach as a non-surgical treatment of genital muscle weakness associated with urinary incontinence (bladder control) and organ (i.e., uterine, bladder) prolapse. Today, they may be referred to as Kegels, or PC exercises, or pelvic floor exercises, with the term PC referring to the pubococcygeus muscle, one of the primary muscles involved in doing these squeezes. We recommend these exercises for every woman at every age.

When should women do these exercises?

▶ Do them regularly, as in 4-5 times per week to enhance genital health, unless instructed otherwise by your healthcare provider;
▶ During pregnancy and after childbirth to facilitate recovery;
▶ In the early stages of organ prolapse to minimize the feeling that 'something is falling out of my vagina;'
▶ In case of injury/neurological deficit to restore muscle tone and function, as instructed by your healthcare provider, and
▶ As an orgasm exercise. Yes, you read that right. The pelvic floor muscles have voluntary and involuntary fibers and are the ones that give you an orgasm with their unique ability to quiver, contract, and squeeze as you are enjoying the culmination of sexual arousal. Many women also instinctively (voluntarily) contract them in a rhythmic manner during intercourse, squeezing the penis to the man's delight.

If you're new to "Kegels," it may be easiest to first try doing them while lying down. As you get stronger, you can do them while sitting and standing. The great thing about Kegels—as we hope you'll discover—is that you can do them anywhere, anytime except while voiding (urinating), and no one will know but you.

This exercise program has two components: fast and slow contractions.

- ▶ Fast contractions: Contract and release, contract and release, with only a momentary pause between each repetition. The goal is to be able to do 30 repetitions in a row.
- ▶ Slow contractions: Contract the muscles and hold for 10 seconds, then release and rest for 10 seconds before starting the next repetition. The goal is to do 10 repetitions in a row.

Patience is key when it comes to Kegels. It will take training to be able to do the above-mentioned number of repetitions, so don't give up! Keep a log of your progress, and you should see great results within 3-6 weeks.

Not sure you're doing them right? Or having trouble feeling if you're doing them at all? Speak to your healthcare provider or to a pelvic floor physical therapist, who can give you direct guidance.

———

Myths and Facts

As we've mentioned, too many women remain ignorant about their own genitals . . . and the abundance of myths, rumors, and misconceptions floating around certainly doesn't help. Consider the following:

- **MYTH: *The vagina is sterile, requiring special cleaning methods to keep it that way.* FACT:** The vagina is not at all sterile, but is host to a multitude of various types of bacteria, which together comprise the vaginal flora that promotes vaginal health. The composition of this flora changes with age, stress, hormone levels, diet, antibiotics, and sexual activity, and is best managed by taking probiotics, so talk to your healthcare provider or to a nutritionist for details and recommendations. As for cleaning the vagina, it is self-cleaning! Meaning, there is no need to douche or do anything else, unless otherwise instructed by a healthcare provider.
- **MYTH: *Things can get lost inside the vagina.*** For some reason, there remains a perception among some women that the vagina

is a long, continuous canal that starts at the genitals and continues deep into the body. So, it's not surprising that women often ask us if anything—a tampon, say—can "get lost" up there. FACT: The vagina is only about 4-4.5 inches (10-12 centimeters) deep. Think of it as a small dead-end tube with an opening only on one end. In the unlikely event that a tampon got "stuck" in there, it can easily be retrieved.

- **MYTH: *Sexual arousal is needed for vaginal penetration.*** FACT: The vagina can always accommodate a penis without the need for sexual arousal. This myth is rooted in the perception that 'if the penis is happily aroused when entering the vagina, then the vagina should be equally happy and aroused when receiving it." But in reality, the vagina is a passive canal that does not change for penetration, whereas the penis must go from flaccid (resting) to sufficiently erect (aroused) to be able to get in. Imagine if a woman needed to be aroused for a gynecologic examination, or for inserting a tampon in her vagina, or during childbirth or vaginal surgery when instruments are placed inside her!

- **MYTH: *Urine comes out of the vagina.*** FACT: Unlike men, for whom the penis serves as both sexual organ and urine outlet, in women, these functions are separate, unless there is an abnormality (fistula), which calls for medical intervention.

- **MYTH: *I don't have a hole.*** FACT: Unless you were born with a specific medical condition (congenital absence of the vagina), you do indeed have a vaginal opening, and are just having some trouble finding it. In the vast majority of cases in which women report that they or their partners "can't find it," the underlying cause is a lack of body-education and/or vaginismus - the inability or great difficulty with vaginal penetrations - a medical condition that is discussed in Chapter Eight.

- **MYTH: *Semen is dangerous to the vagina.*** FACT: Semen, or seminal fluid, is released from the penis when the man ejaculates, and is perfectly safe to the vagina, the mouth, or anywhere else on the body.

- **MYTH: *Tampons are dangerous.*** FACT: Tampons are perfectly safe to use during your period, including at night, as long as you remember to change them regularly. Toxic Shock Syndrome

(TSS), the condition sometimes associated with tampon use, is a complication of bacterial infection caused by staph or strep organisms, and affects men, women, and children. Historically, it was tied to a new tampon called Rely that was manufactured in 1978[1]. However, once the problem was identified and the product removed from the market, returned to be a safe option. That said, it is always a good idea to see your healthcare provider if you experience unexplained fever, rash, or vomiting while using tampons.

———

To Shave or Not to Shave?

The media presents a limited and largely uniform picture of female attractiveness, and this is particularly true when it comes to pornography, where women's pubic areas are almost exclusively depicted as smooth and hairless. In addition to the increased mainstreaming of porn, various TV programs have also been credited with popularizing the notion that a woman is only sexy if her genital area resembles that of a pre-pubescent girl. We do not consider it our place—or anyone's place—to determine how a woman should groom herself in this most personal sphere. As in nearly all facets of the sexual arena, there is no right or wrong here—what matters is that we, as women, feel empowered to make our own choices, whether we're in a relationship or on our own.

———

1. Rely and Toxic Shock Syndrome: A Technological Health Crisis. Accessed January 05, 2015
   http://www.ncbi.nlm.nih.gov/pmc/articles/PMC3238331

(Very) Personal Hygiene

Many of us have been trained since childhood not to talk about anything that has to do with "down there," and, therefore, have never gotten basic information about how to care for our genitals. If we were lucky, we may have had a wise older sister or a female cousin to guide us in these matters. For the rest of us, here's what you need to know to keep your genitals clean, comfortable, and healthy.

- **What's the best way to wash?** We have already established that the vagina is self-cleaning, and that there is no need to wash inside it. For the vulva, apply a bit of hypoallergenic soap in your hand and lightly soap up between your inner and outer lips, separating them with your fingers if necessary; no need to scrub or to use a washcloth, which may be a bit too harsh. To rinse—with warm water, never hot—it's best to use a hand-held attachment to the shower head, which is extremely helpful when it comes to washing inside all the vulva's creases and folds. Alternatively, splash water onto the vulva with a cupped hand, or use a spray bottle filled with warm water, or take a bath, which will rinse your genitals off for you. When you step out of the shower or bath, pat the area dry, and that's it. If you find that your vulva feels dry after bathing, you may apply a thin coat of Aquaphor™ to the skin between the lips as well as to the vaginal opening. One final note: If you enjoy using scented soaps or body washes, it's generally best to save them for other parts of your body. And, if you do find that the soap or bubble bath product you're using is causing an irritation, wash only with water for several days before trying a different product.
- **What should I do about my pubic (genital) hair?** For many of us, this is the eternal question. Women seem to be divided between those who tend to their pubic hair and those who do not. There is absolutely no right or wrong here—either choice is fine as long as it is *your choice*. For those who do choose to tend to their pubic hair, the most popular methods are trimming with scissors, laser removal, waxing, and shaving. Waxing may be minimal, complete (commonly known as a "Brazilian"), or anything in between. If you have

your waxing done by someone else, make sure it is a reputable technician who is in compliance with proper sanitary conditions.

When it comes to shaving, lots of women find that they experience unbecoming raised red bumps. A great tip to prevent this from happening: shave at the sink, rather than in the shower/bath, three hours before or after you bathe, which gives the pores time to close. By the way, this also applies to shaving legs and underarms.

- **What about vaginal odor?** Sadly, many women believe that there is something wrong with the way their genitals smell. And many of them tell us that they are afraid that their partners will not like their scent, or be offended by it and decline intimacy. Some women avoid certain forms of sexual contact, or refrain from sex altogether, because they are concerned that they don't "smell good." Like many other facets of sexual health, this sense of shame can only be combatted with knowledge.

  The simple fact is that the vagina, like the penis, the feet, the underarms, and the nose, ear, and mouth, has its own particular odor. This is a basic physiological fact, and does not mean something is wrong with you! Of course, this can be difficult to keep in mind when there is an entire industry built around the notion that the natural scent of the vagina is something to be masked. Scented douches, deodorants, as well as scented maxi pads and tampons, are heavily marketed to women, with the aim of making money off our collective embarrassment. Before you rush to cover-up your natural fragrance, however, keep in mind that, left alone, the vagina maintains an optimum level of acidity (pH level of 3.8 to 4.5) and a delicate balance of "good" and "bad" bacteria. Applying scented products will easily disrupt this delicate balance and may lead to medical complications, so we strongly advise that you not use any scented products in or near your vagina. Remember: Your natural scent is a sign of a healthy, properly balanced vagina! However, if you remain concerned about odor to the extent that is keeping you from enjoying a stress-free sex life (and your healthcare provider has assured you that your vagina is healthy), it may be worth seeking out a licensed therapist who can help you navigate your underlying feelings of shame or poor self-image.

- **Should I clean up after intercourse?** The answer is that there is no right answer—it completely depends on your personal preference. While some women prefer to rinse off their genitals after intercourse, it is absolutely not necessary, as some of the semen will leak out immediately (the "wet spot"), some will be absorbed by your body, and the rest will be come out later. If rinsing the vagina is your choice, use an emptied douche bottle filled with lukewarm water. *Never use scented or medicinal products unless instructed to do so by your healthcare provider.*
- **Should I urinate after intercourse to prevent a urinary tract infection (UTI)?** There is no clear answer. Some women do not urinate yet never develop a UTI, while many who do still end up with a UTI every time or some of the times. Suggestion: pay attention to your body's susceptibility, and speak with your healthcare provider.

————

Constipation and Sex

While most of us are uncomfortable discussing our bathroom habits and sex lives in the same conversation (let alone discussing them at all!), simple human mechanics mean that the two subjects aren't completely unrelated.

In basic terms, the vaginal canal runs parallel to the urethra (urine tube) that is above it, and to the anal canal that is below it. In other words, the three tubes run parallel to each other, with the vagina being in the middle. So if you are constipated, it is quite possible that penile penetration and/or thrusting will be uncomfortable, or even painful, because of the accumulated feces in the anal canal. For this reason, we recommend staying active and eating a diet rich in fresh fruits and vegetables, which will help to maintain regularity and prevent any bathroom-related problems in the bedroom. If that doesn't help, speak to your healthcare provider.

————

Managing PMS (It's real!)

Every woman will experience her period differently. For some women, the days leading up to our periods pass unnoticed and uneventfully, but for others, the week leading up to menstruation is marked by (often very painful) emotional and physical symptoms caused by hormonal fluctuations—what's known as Premenstrual Syndrome (PMS).

While you may have heard that PMS doesn't *really* exist or that "it's all in your head," the truth is that it is a very real phenomenon. So if you experience any of the following, there's no need to feel embarrassed: You're not the only one!

- "I get such terrible cramps that I have to lie in bed for hours."
- "My migraines/backaches sometimes get so bad that I have to miss work."
- "I get really depressed out of nowhere and find myself crying at the smallest things."
- "My moods are so up and down that I sometimes feel like I'm going a little crazy."
- "I get really sensitive and find myself picking fights with my husband."
- "My skin breaks out, my whole body gets bloated, and I feel like I just look ugly."

The good news is that today there are plenty of tools available to help manage these symptoms—and often, the most effective tools are those we can do by ourselves. Maintaining a healthy diet, rich in fruits and vegetables and exercising regularly has been proven to help, as has stress-relieving, endorphin-releasing activities like yoga and meditation. If the self-help route does not work for you, it may be worth discussing other options with you healthcare provider.

A note on menstruation and sexual activity: For those of us who experience cramping or migraines during our periods, sexual intimacy is typically the last thing we're thinking about, while others of us may restrict sexual activity during menstruation due to religious or cultural considerations. Still others will choose to refrain for aesthetic reasons. However, for many of us our sexual lives may continue uninterrupted during our menstrual cycles. From a medical perspective, there is certainly no right or wrong here, as long as the choice to engage or refrain is your own.

Tampon Tips

If your vagina is chafed or irritated by tampon use, don't despair. Rather than revert back to using sanitary pads, which many of us find bulky, smelly, and uncomfortable, try the following lube trick: Using an empty mini travel container (1 oz or 2 oz size) with a screw-on lid or any such small container, squeeze vaginal lubrication such as KY Jelly™ into it, and carry it with you wherever you go. When you need to insert a tampon, dip its tip into the lube before putting it into the vagina, and make sure to give the tampon an extra push inward so it will rise to its ideal location. To remove a tampon, dip your (clean!) finger into the lube container, insert the lubed finger into the vagina, remove the finger, and glide the tampon out through the now-lubricated lower vagina. Make sure to wash the container regularly.

Leading an Active Lifestyle

Would it surprise you to learn that people who are active—whether it's hitting the gym, walking to work, taking a yoga class, or going hiking on the weekends—typically report having more active and pleasurable sex lives as well? The sense of well-being and positive outlook promoted by exercise are, we would argue, the very foundations of healthy sexuality: When we are active, our bodies work better. It's not a coincidence that the endorphins released during physical activity are similar to those released during orgasm.

Furthermore, there's no question that leading an active lifestyle yields as many benefits for your mental health as it does for your physical health. Study after study links physical exercise to happiness, better memory, and the ability to solve problems. When we work out, our heart, lungs, and endocrine system (to name a few) all benefit. Living in our technologically advanced society, preoccupied with our electronic devices, it's easy to forget that as human beings, we are *designed* to be active. Not only is it our natural state, it is how our bodies heal and mend.

In addition to keeping your body fit and boosting your self-esteem, physical exercise can offer the opportunity to connect with friends or meet new people. If you are in a relationship, it can be a great way to spend time together and bond over a shared interest. And, just in case you think it's too late to get started, research has shown time and time again that exercise benefits people at all ages—well into our eighties.

That said, as women, it is vital that we remember to care for our most intimate areas before, during, and following physical activity.

- Remember to change out of your sweaty workout clothes, whether it's cycling shorts, a bathing suit, or a pair of yoga pants, as soon as possible.
- Launder your workout clothes at the earliest opportunity to avoid bacterial growth.
- Gently wash the vulva using hypoallergenic soap and lukewarm water following physical activity.
- If necessary, apply a barrier ointment such as Aquaphor™ prior to exercise to prevent chafing and irritation.
- If you do experience vulvar irritation during or after your workout, try leaning forward while you urinate; this will help minimizing the burning sensation while the area heals.
- **Swimming:** the chemicals used in swimming pools and the salt in ocean water can cause disruptive vaginal dryness so use a vaginal moisturizer of your choice at bedtime.
- **Running:** if you have recently given birth, keep in mind that your "plumbing" hasn't yet restored itself to its pre-pregnancy state. Running can lead to, or exacerbate, postpartum urinary incontinence, even if you were not struggling with bladder control previously. Also, some women may experience hemorrhoid irritation or pressure. Our suggestions? Make sure to do your Kegel exercises, and opt for other methods of working out while gradually resuming running distance and speed.

- **Cycling:** Whether you're cycling indoors or outdoors, visit a professional bike shop for a good bike fit, wear padded cycling shorts or pants (no underwear needed as they may bunch up and cause irritation), and apply a generous amount of barrier ointment to your vulva to avoid friction.
- And, if you have your period and wear a pad, make sure to change it often, as blood is acidic and can cause additional discomfort.

———

Preparing For Your Gynecologic Exam

When scheduling an elective (non-emergency) gynecologic exam, you may want to follow these tips:

▸ Schedule it for when you are not menstruating.

▸ Bring a list, including the date of your last period, names of prescription medications you are taking, and questions you want to ask. You may also want to bring along a pair of socks to keep your feet warm in the stirrups, and a sanitary pad for afterwards to absorb excess lube or the occasional spotting.

▸ Refrain from using your vagina for 48 hours prior to the exam—sexual intercourse, vaginal preparations, etc.—so that the Pap smear will not be altered by the presence of leftover semen (ejaculate), contraceptive gel/foam, vaginal estrogen, moisturizers, lubricants, etc.

▸ To keep the vagina moist for a more comfortable insertion of the non-lubricated speculum, avoid using tampons for the 48 hours preceding your exam, and take showers only, skipping sitting in a bath, pool, or Jacuzzi, all of which can dry out the vagina.

▸ Contrary to what some women believe, there is absolutely no need to shave your pubic area or your legs before the exam.

———

A Guide to Gynecological Care

Gynecological care varies greatly depending on where you live. In many countries, women see a gynecologist only at the onset of a gynecological problem or when pregnant, while in North America, women are encouraged to have an annual pelvic exam, beginning at the age of 21 or within three years of first having sexual intercourse, whichever comes first[2].

While few women would say they look forward to seeing their gynecologist, it should never be something you dread. It might be helpful to think of a gyno exam like a trip to the dentist—nobody really *wants* to go, but most of us recognize the necessity of preventative and corrective dental care. Hopefully, we care as much about our vaginas as we do about our teeth!

A typical visit to the gynecologist in North America consists of a manual breast exam, followed by a pelvic exam done while you are lying on your back, which includes:

- **A *visual inspection*** of the external genitals, during which your healthcare provider will be on the lookout for any lesions, infections, or trauma.
- **The insertion of a speculum** — a metal or plastic duckbill-like medical instrument - into the vagina. Once inside, it is clicked open for a visual inspection of the vagina itself and for a Pap test. During this phase of the exam, we recommend asking your clinician to hold a mirror near the entrance to your vagina, so you can see inside. It's your body, after all, you should know what it looks like!
- **The Pap test.** Using a tiny brush, the clinician will collect cells from the cervix and the area around it for the detection of abnormalities and cancer. The test is quick and painless; you may feel nothing, or a faint pinching sensation. You will be fine afterwards, though some women may spot a bit. To visualize the Pap test, think of a throat culture that it is done to the cervix (thankfully, without a gag reflex to worry about). Historical trivia: do

2. ACOG Practice Advisory on Annual Pelvic Examination Recommendations. Accessed January 05, 2015. http://www.acog.org/About-ACOG/News-Room/Statements-and-Advisories/2014/ACOG-Practice-Advisory-on-Annual-Pelvic-Examination-Recommendations

you know what the word Pap stands for? It is short for Georgios Nikolaou Papanicolaou, a twentieth-century Greek physician who was a pioneer in cytopathology and early cancer detection.

- **A digital (manual) exam.** The clinician will insert his or her finger/s into the vagina while pressing the other hand against the lower abdomen to feel for tenderness, swelling, or other abnormalities. Some clinicians may simultaneously insert one finger into the vagina and another into the rectal canal to get a better feel for the area, or to collect mucosal sampling for anal cancer screening.

Breast Awareness

Because most breast cancers are self-diagnosed, women in the West were once widely encouraged to perform monthly breast exams on themselves. However, a study published in 2014[3] asserts that self-examination has been proven to have no effect on mortality from breast cancer, and as a result, guidelines have evolved: In place of monthly self-exams, women in the U.S. are now encouraged to develop what is called "breast self-awareness," meaning a familiarity with how their breasts look and feel, and to be mindful of any changes, which should be reported to their healthcare provider.

A routine gyno exam should not hurt, should not cause distress, and should not feel belittling in any way. If it does hurt, to the point of being impossible to complete, or causes you great emotional distress, it's possible

---

3. Mark K, Temkin SM, Terplan M. Breast Self-Awareness: The Evidence Behind the Euphemism. Obstetrics & Gynecology. April 2014. Volume 123; issue 4; pp 734-736. http://www.ncbi.nlm.nih.gov/pubmed/24785598

that you may be suffering from vaginismus. Sadly, it's not unusual for women to report that they struggle with the physical or with the emotional component of the exam, or with both.

From an anatomical standpoint, the key to a physically comfortable exam is to minimize your reflexive response of bracing. What do we mean by that? Well, for many women, the reflexive reaction during a gynecologic exam is to tighten up the pelvic floor (PC muscles) as the clinician is about to "go in." Unfortunately, the physical fact is that the more you tighten up, the more discomfort you will feel. We recommend that as you lie there, heels in stirrups, rather than think about the exam, focus on keeping your legs open and your vaginal muscles relaxed. Keeping your breathing at meditation rate, picture your vagina welcoming the penetration. If you can do that, the exam should be quick and painless.

From an emotional standpoint, some women report struggling with one or more of the following:

- "I don't feel comfortable bringing my most intimate questions to my healthcare provider."
- "My doctor doesn't listen to me."
- "I wonder if a female clinician would have made the experience better for me . . ."
- "My doctor doesn't explain what he/she is doing during the exam."
- "When I bring a specific concern to my physician, she brushes it off like it's nothing."
- "My doctor has told me, 'It's all in your head.'"
- "I am a lesbian and I feel that my sexual care and needs are not being addressed."
- "I wish my doctor would have started the conversation (about sex, relationships, abuse) because I am too embarrassed . . ."
- "I have vaginismus—how do I tell them not to force an exam on me? I would rather discuss the problem and treatment options."
- "Am I the only one who is nervous about the exam?"

Sound familiar? We like to remind our patients that selecting a healthcare provider is a choice, especially nowadays when we are more informed than ever about our bodies, having done our share of Internet research and having prepared ourselves with good questions. All of us have the right to a mutually respectful dialogue with our healthcare providers. If you have a gut feeling that something is not right—that your concerns are not being taken seriously, that you aren't encouraged to ask questions, trust your instinct! Remember: It's your body and your health—you have the right to choose your medical guide.

Lying on your back with your heels in stirrups and your legs open is not an experience women relish, but avoiding pelvic exams only keeps us ignorant and fearful. Remember: Knowledge is power, and power is control. So if you're overdue for your annual exam, or if you have a nagging vaginal concern that you've been trying to ignore, make an appointment today. Chances are you'll feel relieved—and even gratified—knowing that you are taking responsibility for your health and well-being.

_____

What If I Have An Abnormal Pap?

So, your Pap smear results came back "inconclusive" or "suspicious," and you were told you need to repeat the test in several months. Of course, you're nervous, worried, maybe even convinced that you have cancer. While these feelings are perfectly understandable, we highly recommend taking a moment to breathe deeply. An abnormal Pap test need not be the end of the world. In reality, false-positive results are not unusual and may be due to laboratory errors or to the presence of blood, mucus, inflammation, semen, spermicidal jelly, or other vaginal preparations, all of which can alter the result. If the abnormalities require close scrutiny, your healthcare provider will likely recommend repeating the Pap smear in three months, unless the findings call for more aggressive intervention. What can you do to minimize false-positive results in the future? Leave your vagina alone for 48 hours prior to your exam, giving it a chance to self-cleanse of any residue. In the meantime, try to stay as calm as possible until you do the repeat test—it may very well come back negative and normal.

_____

An Infection or an Irritation?

If you're feeling a burning and/or itching sensation in your vagina and/or vulva, including burning during intercourse or urination, your first thought is probably that you have an infection, right? Well, guess what? Often, what many of us assume to be an infection is, in fact, not an infection at all but merely an *irritation*. Learning to distinguish between an irritation and an infection is very important in order to avoid unnecessary worry and intervention. (A reminder: if you're in doubt, or if the persists for more than a few days, seek medical advice.)

Vaginal irritation can be caused by any one or more of the following, and typically resolve on their own within a short time:

- Wearing sweaty workout clothes or a wet bathing suit for an extended period of time.
- Engaging in a long and sweaty sexual act.
- Sleeping in heavy pajamas or an overly warm blanket.
- Wearing stockings in hot and humid conditions.
- Sitting for many hours on a vinyl chair, which provides no air circulation for your bottom.
- Excessive sweating between skin folds, i.e. vulva, groin, or under breasts.
- Wearing tight jeans that rub or aggravate the area.
- Not changing one's sanitary pads frequently enough.
- Increased sugar intake, including not only processed foods, but sugary fruits as well (grapes, melons, raisins, etc.).
- Menopausal changes, including hot flashes, vaginal dryness, vaginal chafing from intercourse, spotting after intercourse, clitoral irritation.
- Prolonged or repeated use of antibiotics, which negatively affects the protective function of "good" bacteria in the vagina.
- Engaging in intercourse past one's comfort, resulting in vaginal hot spots, vaginal dryness, or micro-tears of the vestibule, also known as the "6 o'clock spot." If this applies to you, keep in mind that it is your body—and your right to ask your partner to withdraw if you're uncomfortable. It's also worth applying a

lubricating gel inside the vagina prior to intercourse—and reapplying as soon as you feel your vaginal skin beginning to chafe.
- Vaginal chafing upon inserting or removing a tampon.
- Urethral chafing. (See below).

As a woman, chances are you'll experience a vaginal infection at some point in your life. And, some of us may be faced with recurring infections that can affect our physical comfort, our sexual practices, even our self-esteem.

How you treat an infection will depend in large part on the country and culture you live in. In some places, vaginal infections are treated holistically—with dietary changes, homemade remedies, or herbal preparations, while in others, such as the U.S. and U.K., infections are typically treated with prescription or over-the-counter medications. Either way, there is increasing awareness among Western women that relatively simple changes in diet and personal habits can be effective tools in preventing a problem in the first place. That said, some infections require immediate medical attention, so it is worth visiting your healthcare provider to determine the appropriate course of action.

The following is a short infection primer:

- **Vaginal yeast infection**—Yeast is a naturally occurring organism that usually lives in happy cohabitation with other organisms in the vaginal ecosystem. A yeast infection occurs when there is a breakdown in this careful balance, caused by any number of factors, including unaddressed vaginal dryness, increased sugar or alcohol intake, antibiotics, sweaty and moist conditions (see earlier in this chapter), a new male sexual partner—even stress. Symptoms vary widely, and may include thick discharge with an unpleasant odor; itchiness; or a mild to strong burning sensation. To say yeast infections are common is an understatement. For treatment, some women will try holistic remedies, some will opt for self-treatment with over-the-counter preparations, including prescription-strength vaginal suppositories or creams administered via applicator, only seeking medical advice if those don't do the trick, while others will schedule a medical appointment right away. It's very important that you tell your healthcare provider if you cannot use or afraid to use a vaginal applicator due to vaginismus or any other reason, so that an alternative treatment, such as oral medication, can be prescribed. It's also important to refrain from sexual intercourse while undergoing treatment. Lastly, your vagina will become quite dry following treatment, so use as much lubrication as is necessary to make sexual intercourse comfortable for the first two to three weeks after your infection's cleared up.

- **Urinary tract infection (UTI):** The causes of UTIs are wide-ranging, from having vaginal intercourse with a new partner, to pregnancy, to being menopausal. Symptoms include the frequent urge to urinate without much urine being released; pain or burning upon urination; lower-abdomen pain; and cloudy or discolored urine. UTIs are usually treated with oral antibiotics, which kill the "bad" bacteria. Some women will need more than one course of antibiotics to eradicate the infection; some women will experience recurring UTIs and will need antibiotics every few weeks. Unfortunately, being non-discriminating, the antibiotics also kill the "good" bacteria—the protective organisms that live in the gut and the vagina. The typical result: a vagina that is dry, itchy, and less elastic, which makes it more sensitive to stretching and to chafing, as well as to developing a yeast infection. So if you develop these conditions after taking antibiotics for a UTI or any other bodily infection, it's worth discussing with your healthcare provider, who can help you choose a course of restorative care, which should include probiotics.

- **Bacterial vaginosis**—An imbalance in vaginal bacteria with no one specific cause. Its main symptom is a heavy, foul-smelling discharge. If you have persistent discharge that fits this description, you'll need to pay a visit to your healthcare provider, who is likely to prescribe antibiotics.

Urethral Chafing

Urethral chafing is a form of vaginal irritation that is so common—and so misunderstood—that it deserves its own section. In fact, while few women have ever heard of this, it is one of the most frequently occurring conditions we see in our practice. Because its symptoms are so similar to those that arise with a UTI (burning; urinary urgency), it remains misdiagnosed in untold numbers of women. The result? Unnecessary medications for an infection that does not exist, and lots of women avoiding sex because it is simply too painful.

So what is urethral chafing? As was mentioned at the beginning of this chapter, the lower urethra runs like a tube in the ceiling of the vagina, while from above it is bound by the underside of the pubic bone. This alignment gives the lower urethra a soft floor (the vagina) and a hard ceiling (the pubic bone). Functionally speaking, whenever anything goes into the vagina, it "rubs" against the floor of the urethra, which is covered by fatty, estrogenic tissue that can be likened to protective bubble wrapping. However, when breakdowns occur, the urethra will make its discomfort known by way of urinary urgency, burning, and irritation. Much as it may feel like a UTI, it is not. Urethral chafing, which can also be thought of as an "upset urethra," may be caused by one or more of the following:

- Compromised estrogen, as in the case of menopause.
- Insufficient lubrication during sexual intercourse.
- Inserting a tampon into a dry vagina.
- Having recently completed treatment for a vaginal infection, before the "good" bacteria, natural lubrication, and elasticity are restored.
- Prolonged sexual intercourse that rubs the urethra beyond its tolerance.
- Repeated sexual intercourse within a short time frame.
- Intercourse with a penis that is thicker than average.
- Use of a dilator or a dildo without added lubrication when needed.
- Sexual intercourse with a man who has Peyronie's disease (when the curvature of the penis is pointed upward).

- Anxiety, because it causes dryness (vagina, mouth, eyes), and reflexively tightens the pelvic floor muscles, thus narrowing the vagina and subjecting the urethra to stronger friction.

The solution? Give your urethra a vacation! In other words, let it heal without interruption by avoiding the activity that caused the irritation in the first place. We also suggest drinking Stinging Nettle tea, a urinary strengthener that will aid with recovery. Our recommended dose is three tea bags per day, prepared per instructions, then diluted to any consistency and drank at desired temperature. If these steps do not resolve the irritation quickly, you may need further intervention, so be mindful of the situation and seek medical advice.

A Guide to Vaginal Products

Today, there are so many vaginal preparations—creams, lotions, gels, lubricants, and suppositories—available at the local pharmacy and online, all aimed at promoting vaginal health. But how do you know which one to use, and when? If you're confused, you're not alone, so let's sort it out.

▸ **Vaginal moisturizers**—The equivalent of hand or body lotion, vaginal moisturizers add moisture to dry vaginal tissue, typically by mimicking the chemical makeup of the vaginal flora. What are common causes of vaginal dryness? Excessive hygiene, menopause, cancer treatment, certain medications, insufficient hydration, dry heating in the winter, and spending time in a pool, Jacuzzi, or ocean. Over-the-counter vaginal moisturizers (available without a prescription) such as Replens®, RepHresh®, Vagisil®, Luvena®, and Hyalo Gyn®, designed to be used at bedtime, will work their magic inside your vagina while you sleep. *An important note: Vaginal moisturizers are chemically made as a treatment to nourish the vagina and thus are not suitable for sexual activities*

- *Vaginal lubricants*—These are used to ease vaginal penetration, to minimize friction during sexual intercourse, or when using a dildo. They vary in consistency and ingredients—water-based, silicone-based, petroleum-based—and are available in different formulations—liquids, gels, and suppositories—even in different flavors. You may need to experiment a bit to find the product that works best for you and does not cause irritation or allergic reactions.
- *Vaginal estrogen*— A hormonal replacement preparation for when natural estrogen is depleted, such as in menopause, after suppression therapy for fibroids, endometriosis, or cancer, or after removal of ovaries. Introducing estrogen into the vagina will help to restore vaginal tissue and elasticity, as well as reduce the feeling of dryness and discomfort, and prevent the associated urinary frequency and urgency. Vaginal estrogen is available by prescription and comes in different forms, including creams (Estrace, Premarin), tablets (Vagifem), vaginal rings (Estring), and bio-identical formulations. To figure out which best suits your needs, discuss the various options with your healthcare provider. *An important note: Vaginal estrogen is not designed for sexual activities; for that purpose, use vaginal lubricants.*

What You Need To Know About Sexually Transmitted Infections

Sometimes referred to as sexually transmitted diseases (STDs), sexually transmitted infections (STIs) are infections that are passed from person to person through a range of sexual activities—and not only through intercourse, as some people believe. STIs don't care if you're single or married, gay or straight, rich or poor. And, they don't care if you're having oral sex, anal sex, or vaginal sex. They can be passed from man to woman, woman to man, man to man or woman to woman, without regard for level of sexual experience or duration of your relationship.

In other words, STIs are incredibly prevalent . . . so if you've suffered one in the past, are dealing with one now, or suspect you might be, rest assured you are not alone.

The following are the most commonly occurring STIs:

- **Chlamydia**—frequently transmitted to women by men who have no idea they are carriers because they are asymptomatic. In women, symptoms may include vaginal burning, particularly during urination. If left untreated, Chlamydia may lead to infertility or other complications.
- **Genital warts**—caused by the human papillomavirus (HPV). Highly contagious flesh-color bumps or cauliflower-like growths that may appear on the vulva, around the anus, and/or inside the rectum and vagina.
- **Genital herpes**—typically caused by Herpes Simplex type 2, and easily passed through oral, vaginal, or anal sex with an infected partner. Take notice: oral herpes (cold sores which appear on the lips or mouth), typically caused by Herpes Simplex type 1, are just as contagious as genital herpes—and can be transmitted to the genitals via oral sex or by a hand that touched the sore on the mouth, then touched the genitals —so if you or your partner is having an outbreak, stay away from each other until it has been properly treated and the outbreak is resolved.
- **Gonorrhea**—some women may experience unusual vaginal discharge or pelvic pain, while some may have such mild symptoms that the infection goes unnoticed. Others may confuse it with a yeast infection and treat it as such. Untreated, Gonorrhea can affect the heart and joints, leading to serious health problems.
- **Syphilis**—because this infection develops in stages, it may be asymptomatic for a while, or present itself with sores or a rash on the hands or feet, fever, a general ill feeling, and/or joint and muscle pain. Once present in epidemic-like numbers, it is now easily treated with penicillin.
- **Human immunodeficiency virus (HIV)** is the virus that causes AIDS, a condition that weakens the immune system and allows

life-threatening opportunistic infection and cancers to thrive. It is contracted through unprotected sex with an infected partner, or needle sharing.

- **Human Papillomavirus (HPV)**—The most common STI. There are many strains of related viruses in this group that specifically affect the genitals. In most cases HPV will resolve on its own without causing any problems; sometimes, though, it is the cause for genital warts (see above) or cancer of the cervix. While the vaccine may protect against most genital warts and most cases of cervical cancer, it is not a full protection and, vaccinated women still need to undergo screening.

In most cases, the earlier you treat an STI, the better. If you suspect that you have an infection, we recommend seeing your healthcare provider immediately, so that you can begin treatment as soon as possible.

The good news is that the risk for contracting an STI can be greatly reduced by practicing safe sex—using a condom or dental dam for vaginal, anal, and oral sex (for more information on dental dams, see Chapter Four)—and by insisting that both you *and* your partner get tested for the entire STI panel, and show each other the results.

So why are STIs still so prevalent? Because, in addition to being highly contagious, they are often invisible—meaning that a person may have an STI but not have any symptoms. It is very common for an individual to be unaware of being infected in the first place, while others may simply be reluctant to let their partners know the truth. That is why it is absolutely mandatory to use condoms in each and every sexual encounter, unless you are in a committed long-term relationship and both of you have already tested negative.

Sadly, many women are still hesitant to bring up the subject of condoms with prospective partners, believing that "it will upset him" or "he's such a clean-cut, responsible guy, there's no way he could have an STI." As we know all too well, however, the honor system doesn't always work. And so, we urge our patients—and all women—to overcome any embarrassment or apprehension, and **have the talk**. If you are still uncomfortable broaching the subject, it may be worth considering whether it makes sense for you to engage sexually with someone with whom you cannot talk honestly. (We discuss this subject at greater length in Chapter Three: Where are the condoms?)

When to See Your Healthcare Provider

In general, we encourage women to seek medical advice any time they notice something out of the ordinary. In addition, we recommend a visit to a healthcare provider if you experience any of the following:

▸ The absence of a period

▸ An irregular period

▸ Bleeding outside of your regular cycle

▸ Exceptionally heavy period

▸ Severe mood swings

▸ Unmanageable Premenstrual Syndrome (PMS)

▸ Sustained weakness during your period

▸ Unusual vaginal discharge or odor

▸ Itching

▸ Skin lesions, including pimples, sores, rash, peeling skin

▸ Sudden pain (with or without sexual activity)

▸ Swelling or distension of abdomen

▸ Burning with urination

▸ Blood in the urine

▸ Bleeding when in menopause

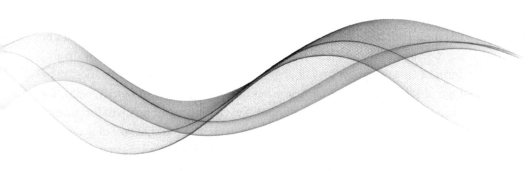

Chapter Two

The Fertile Years

Contraception, Pregnancy, and Beyond

A s women, negotiating our fertility can sometimes feel like a full-time job, with challenges and opportunities, good days and bad. Whether we're researching the various contraception options or attempting to navigate the ever-expanding range of fertility treatments, we may sometimes feel like we are making our way through an endless maze of complicated—and sometimes conflicting—information. While we will not attempt in these pages to provide a comprehensive account of all the potential factors surrounding fertility (which would require a book onto itself), our aim in these pages is to address the impact that our fertility has on our lives, particularly when it comes to the sexual sphere, and to help you make the choices that are right for you.

Contraceptive Options

If you're sexually active and pregnancy is not part of your immediate plan, then using contraception is a must. Today, there are more options than ever before, though there is still no perfect solution. Each method has its pros and cons, and there can be wide variance in reliability and effectiveness. We like to remind our patients that finding the right method of contraception can be a process of trial and error. It's also worth keeping in mind that the "right" form of contraception may change along with your life circumstances. The type of birth control we choose when we're single and in our twenties, for example, may not be what we choose if we're in a relationship of longstanding in our forties. It's also important to keep in mind that you may need to experiment with different types of birth control if you find that you're having adverse side-effects to the one you're currently using. What remains important is to be aware of your options and to find the one that works best for *you*.

Broadly speaking, there are four types of birth control: mechanical/barrier, natural, hormonal, and surgical (sometimes called "sterilization").

Mechanical/barrier contraceptive options include:

- **Male condom**—a thin latex or non-latex cap that the man places over his penis prior to intercourse.
- Female condom—a soft, flexible pouch that the woman inserts into her vagina prior to intercourse.
- **Diaphragm**—a latex cap that the woman inserts into her vagina, along with spermicidal jelly, prior to intercourse.
- **Vaginal Contraceptive Film (VCF)**—a tissue-thin spermicide-releasing film that a woman places deep into her vagina prior to intercourse.
- **Spermicide**—a sperm-destroying agent that may come in the form of a cream, gel, foam, or suppository, which a woman inserts prior to intercourse.
- **Intrauterine Device (IUD)**—a small, non-medicated metal device inserted into the woman's uterus by a health care provider. The IUD can remain in the woman's body for many years, depending on the brand.

Note: Male and female condoms are the only forms of contraception that also help to prevent sexually transmitted infections

Natural contraceptive options include:

- **The rhythm method**—sometimes referred to as natural family planning or the fertility awareness method, this entails keeping track of the woman's menstrual cycle and avoiding intercourse during the days she is considered most fertile. (This method may also include "pulling out," meaning that during so-called fertile days, the man withdraws his penis from the woman's vagina right before ejaculation, which is not a reliable form of birth control.) This method may also include the use of ovulation kits and/or the monitoring of body temperature (see below) and vaginal mucous.
- **Basal body temperature method**—measuring one's basal body temperature is a method of predicting when ovulation takes place—and therefore, when a woman is most fertile—so that she can avoid intercourse accordingly. Alternately, some women use this method to predict their most fertile days when they are trying to conceive. Basal body thermometers, which measure a woman's body temperature down to the decimal point, are widely available in drugstores.

Hormonal contraceptive options include:

- **Oral contraception**, commonly known as "the Pill"—a hormone medication taken daily.
- **"The patch"** (also known by its brandname Ortho Evra)—a hormone-releasing adhesive that a woman affixes to her upper arm or elsewhere on her body once a week.
- **Vaginal ring** (also known by its brandname NuvaRing)—a plastic ring inserted into the vagina once a month that releases estrogen and progestin.
- **Injections** (also known by its brandname Depo-Provera)—a hormone shot that is administered by a health care provider every three months.
- **Contraceptive gel**—a hormone-releasing gel that a woman rubs onto her skin daily.
- **Long-acting reversible contraceptive options:**

- **Hormonal IUD**—a small metal device inserted into the woman's uterine cavity, where it releases progestin. The IUD remains in the woman's body until she decides to have it removed, or it is about to lose it potency. It is similar to the IUD mentioned above; the difference is that it actually releases hormones.
- **Implant**—placed under the skin by a healthcare provider, contraceptive implants release fertilization-inhibiting hormones for a period of up to three years

Surgical options include:

- **Vasectomy** (for the male partner)—a surgical procedure which prevents sperm from being released when a man ejaculates. In some cases, a vasectomy can be surgically reversed.
- **Tubal ligation** (commonly referred to as having one's "tubes tied")—a surgical procedure in which a woman's fallopian tubes are blocked, tied, or cut, preventing the possibility of the eggs traveling to the uterus and being fertilized. Although intended as a permanent sterilization, in some cases, tubal ligation reversal surgery may be possible.

A Word On Emergency Contraception

In an ideal world, we find the form of birth control that works best for us and use it regularly as directed. In the real world, however, things don't always go according to plan, which means that there may be occasions when we find ourselves having unprotected sex. This could be because we neglected to take a pill, because we were too afraid or embarrassed to bring up the subject of birth control with our partner, or because our method of contraception failed (as in the proverbial "the condom broke").

Regardless of the cause, there may be times when we need emergency contraception—meaning contraception that can be used up to 72 or 120 hours *after* intercourse. The most common form of emergency contraception is hormone-releasing pills, often referred to as "the morning-after pill." In most countries, including the US and the UK, women over the age of sixteen can obtain the pill at most major pharmacies without a prescription. Another option is the copper-T IUD, which can prevent pregnancy if inserted within several days after unprotected sex. While both methods are effective emergency contraceptive measures, they are not recommended as an ongoing form of birth control.

———

Deciding what kind of birth control to use is a very personal decision, which, ideally, takes your personality, lifestyle, and future goals into account. Regardless of whether you make the decision on your own or with a partner, it's worth asking yourself the following questions:

- Do I plan on becoming pregnant in the near future, and if so, do I want a form of birth control that's easily reversible?
- Can my partner be counted on to take care of contraception?
- Will my health insurance cover the cost?
- Do I have ongoing access to a healthcare provider?
- Do I need ongoing, longterm contraception or do I only need contraception on an occasional basis?
- Do I have enough information about potential side effects?
- Can I remember to take my medication daily, or does it make more sense for me to opt for a method that I don't need to think about every day?
- Do I prefer to have spontaneous sex or do I like to plan it?
- Have I had any adverse reactions to any forms of birth control in the past?

What You Need To Know About the Pill

Despite what magazine advertisements might lead you to believe, oral contraception does not equal a glamorous night out at a party, nor is it the magic bullet that will open the door to sexual bliss and personal freedom. While "the Pill" may be a sensible birth control option for some women, it is not by any means for everyone. Because the Pill is available only by prescription and because it must be taken at about the same time every single day, it is important to consider **a.** whether you have ongoing access to a healthcare provider, and **b.** whether you have healthcare coverage that will help to cover the monthly expense, and **c.** whether you are the kind of person who is able to remember to take your Pill at the appointed time. (It's okay if you're not! Consistency is not everyone's strong suit. For some women, this is a dealbreaker; others devise ways to remind themselves, such as setting a daily alarm on their smartphone.)

The Pill is available in different hormone combinations; depending on which kind you are taking, you may experience one or more of the following side effects:

- nausea
- bloating
- cramping
- non-menstrual bleeding or spotting
- irritability
- mood swings
- depression
- yeast infection
- decreased sexual desire
- weight gain

While these symptoms may abate with time for some, other women see little or no improvement. If you are experiencing any of these, or other symptoms, we recommend discussing your concerns with your healthcare provider, who can help you determine whether it makes sense to try another type of Pill with a different hormone dosage, or if you prefer to explore other contraception options.

Sex and Pregnancy

Before the Sperm Meets the Egg

Before pregnancy is on the table, sex can serve any number of roles in our life: it can be a source of pleasure and fun, a way to connect to another person, an opportunity to deepen a relationship, a chance to explore and learn about our own desires and preferences. When we're trying to conceive, however, intercourse takes on a whole new dimension: Will this time be the time? Will it happen right away? What if I'm infertile—or what if my partner is?

In addition to any apprehension you may be experiencing, there is no shortage of myths floating around about how to conceive . . . and plenty of unsolicited advice as well. No, you don't need to lie with your legs up in the air following sex . . . sperm has a very effective mechanism for reaching the cervix on its own. However, there are steps you can take to increase your chances of getting pregnant sooner rather than later, beginning with taking care of your own health, mental as well as physical. Scientific studies have proven that the more anxiety a woman has, the less chance she has of conceiving. Aside from fertility issues, we all know that anxiety and sex make unhappy bedfellows. So do whatever you can to keep your anxiety levels in check (easier said than done for some of us!), whether that means finding a relaxing yoga class, doing daily breathing exercises, taking up meditation, or seeking psychotherapy.

Of course, the first step you'll need to take when trying to conceive is discontinuing the use of contraception. If you have been using a barrier method such as a condom or a diaphragm, all you need to do is stop using it. If, however, you've been on the Pill or another form of hormonal contraception, you will need to discuss discontinuing usage with your healthcare provider. (Some women are able to get pregnant immediately upon discontinuing use of the Pill, while it may take others several months before they become fertile again.)

Once you're off contraception, it's a good idea to begin keeping track of your ovulation cycle. Given that most women don't know their exact day of ovulation, it's recommended to have intercourse every other day for ten days, counting from the last day of your period. It is important to remember that the ovaries take turns ovulating—one month it is the right ovary, and the next month is the left ovary—so you may want to give yourself nine to twelve months of trying to conceive before seeking fertility counseling. It is not recommended to engage in intercourse daily when trying to conceive, as this can deplete sperm.

Other things you may want to start thinking about include . . .

- Eating a healthful, nutritionally balanced diet.
- Exercising regularly.
- Checking with your healthcare provider about any medications you may be taking, including anti-depressant or anti-anxiety medications.
- Quitting smoking.
- Reducing alcohol intake if you're a regular drinker.
- Taking a prenatal vitamin (in addition to filling in any missing gaps in your diet, prenatal vitamins contain folic acid, which is vital to the health of your fetus).
- Undergoing genetic counseling as needed.
- Ensuring that your partner is in good health and taking care of him - or herself - as well.

Kids: To Have or Not To Have

Generations ago, there was no such question as "Do I want to have kids?" If you were a woman of childbearing age, it was simply something that was taken for granted. Over the past several decades, however, having children has become less of a given in the Western world and instead has come to be seen as a conscious decision made by couples or, increasingly, by single women who are interested in becoming parents on their own. Because having a child is likely to be one of the most (if not *the* most) significant decisions of one's life, with incalculable emotional, logistical, and financial demands, we applaud the development to treat it as such.

That said, there's no question that the pressure to have children can be enormous, particularly if you come from a religious family or traditional culture. Even so, we like to remind our patients that it's your body, your life, and your decision. While there are plenty of wonderful reasons to bring a child into your life, there are also plenty of not-so-good reasons—like wanting to make your mother happy by giving her a grandchild or hoping that a baby will somehow save a relationship. So rather than allowing baby-making to happen by accident (oops!), we encourage women to do an inventory of their physical and mental health, family support system, and financial resources before taking on the challenge.

If you have a partner, we suggest taking stock of the state of your relationship and targeting areas for improvement; in spite of what many of us may want to believe, not only will having a baby not solve any relationship problems, the stresses of parenthood are likely to exacerbate them. For this reason, we encourage having a frank, honest discussion with your partner (or with a trusted friend, if you are considering embarking on parenthood on your own) about how a baby would fit into your lives. Some questions to consider include: Will your healthcare plan cover the costs of prenatal care and childbirth? Will your job provide maternity leave? Will your partner's job provide parental leave? What kind of childcare arrangements are available to you?

While the decision to forgo parenthood (or put it off until a time when you feel more ready) is becoming more socially acceptable, communicating with family members about it can still be fraught, and may provoke criticism. In such cases, the best you may be able to do is to draw clear boundaries and remember that at the end of the day, the choice whether—or when—to have a child must ultimately be your own.

During pregnancy

Once upon a time, it was thought that sexual activity and pregnancy did not mix. Today, we know that unless medically indicated otherwise, there is no reason why we can't enjoy our sexuality even as our bodies take on the role of growing a new life. Of course, as our bodies change throughout the nine months, so will our sex lives. But how our sex lives are affected varies dramatically from woman to woman.

For some of us, pregnancy is a time of heightened desire—a time when we feel sexy and beautiful, lit from within with the famous "pregnancy glow"—and a time in which we crave sexual intimacy with our partners (particularly during the second trimester, after any first trimester nausea has likely abated, but before the final trimester, when we may simply be too exhausted).[4] For others, pregnancy is defined primarily by physical discomfort—queasiness, vomiting, headaches, fatigue, backaches, urinary incontinence, the list goes on . . . Combined with anxiety about the upcoming birth (not to mention anxiety about parenthood), it's no wonder pregnancy can make us feel anything but sexy. While some of our patients report having experienced the best sex of their lives during those nine months—helped, no doubt, by raised estrogen levels and plenty of natural vaginal lubrication—others are eager for the months to pass quickly so they can get back to their regular old selves. As one of our patients put it, "I just can't wait to feel normal again."

Whether you experience pregnancy as a time of sexual contentment or sexual indifference (or if, like many women, you alternate between the two) depends on a wide range of factors—from whether or not the pregnancy was planned to your physical health to your relationship status. Of course, when it comes to sex, it takes two to tango. So if you are in a relationship, your partner's feelings about the pregnancy will inevitably come into play. While some men (and women) find a woman's pregnant body to be an incredible turn-on—not to mention proof of their virility—others may feel hesitant about resuming the sexual relationship. "Will I hurt the baby?" is a common concern for many men when it comes to intercourse during pregnancy (the answer, by the way, is a definitive "no"—the baby is safely ensconced in the uterus), but your partner may also have less tangible concerns: He may be feeling left out of all the changes going on (after all, they're happening in *your* body, not his), or he may be worried about feeling like a third wheel once the baby actually arrives, or he may feel unsure about how to touch you—even if you've been together for years.

---

4. In religious communities that prohibit sexual contact during and following menstruation, pregnancy offers the freedom of an uninterrupted sexual relationship.

If you and your partner are on the same page, that's great. If not, some gentle negotiating may be in order. Rather than risk miscommunication and hurt feelings during this sensitive time, we encourage couples to set aside a time to talk about the subject without any distractions. Let your partner know how you're feeling about your changing body and your relationship. Don't be afraid to tell him/her what you want (as in, "I'm feeling like a rhinoceros. I need you to show me that you still find me attractive")—most likely, your partner will find it helpful. Ask him/her what his/her concerns and feelings are and see if you can strike a compromise ("I'm not in the mood to have intercourse, but I'd be open to being sexual in other ways").

Remember that ultimately, it's your choice whether and how you want to be intimate. If and when you're ready, here are some tips:

- **Prioritize your own comfort.** Your body is changing, so your tried-and-true repertoire may not be feasible at the moment. Let your own comfort be your guide, and let your partner know what's going on. For example, if your breasts are particularly sensitive—a common occurrence during pregnancy—remind your partner to touch them extra gently (or not at all).
- **Try new positions.** Adaptability is key during this time, especially when it comes to intercourse. As your pregnancy progresses—and your belly expands—certain positions, such as missionary, may no longer be possible. So use pregnancy as an excuse to mix things up. Many couples find that woman-on-top, side-by-side (spooning), and "doggie style" (the man entering the woman from behind while she is on all fours) are the most comfortable during pregnancy.
- **Explore the Sexual Menu** (see Chapter 4). If intercourse is not possible for medical reasons—or even if it is—that is no reason to forgo sexual intimacy. Once again, pregnancy can be an opportunity to explore new avenues of pleasure, from oral sex to sensual foot rubs.

After childbirth

Congratulations! You've managed to get through pregnancy, and now you're holding your long-awaited bundle of joy in your arms. With a newborn keeping you busy at all hours of the day and night, and a body that is still recovering (whether from a vaginal birth or Caesarean), sex is undoubtedly nowhere to be seen on your to-do list. With all the focus on the baby, it can be all too easy to forget that the first weeks (and months) following birth are a time of physical, emotional, and mental adjustment for us not just as mothers, but as women. During the first six to eight weeks following birth, your body—and mind!—need time to realign themselves as your hormones return to pre-pregnancy levels and your body restores itself to pre-pregnancy state.

No matter how much you're enjoying your adorable new addition, there's no question that the postpartum period is a time of major transition: Not only are you acclimating to life with a newborn (whether this is your first child or your fifth), you are also adjusting to shifts in your mood, your relationships, your household arrangements, even your finances. Though you may be feeling happy, you may also be feeling any number of other, less socially acceptable, emotions—anxious, fearful, overwhelmed, or just plain sad. Like many women, you may be alternating between profound joy and profound distress. And often, the pressure to pretend that we are not experiencing any difficult feelings can make them all the harder to manage. If feelings of isolation and despair persist, you may be experiencing postpartum depression.

While you are showering attention on your little one, it is vital that you also find a way to give some attention to yourself—even if all you can manage at first is a nap or a long, hot shower. As women, we are often hesitant to ask for what we need from others, but if ever there is a time to reach out for help, this is it! If you have a partner, let him or her know how they can help, whether it's taking the baby for certain hours of the day (and night!), making dinner, folding laundry, or booking you a massage. Don't be afraid to call upon close friends, neighbors, siblings, parents or in-laws to pitch in so that you can get some much-needed time to yourself.

It's no wonder that, if you think of sex at all during this time, it may be only to wonder, will I ever want to have sex again? As one new mother we know reported telling her husband, "Call me in ten years!" If this sounds familiar, you're not alone. A lack of interest in sex is a totally natural, normal, and necessary part of the recovery process. Just because you're not craving sexual intimacy, however, doesn't mean there's no room for other kinds of intimacy. A hug, a back rub, or even—gasp!—a dinner out can go a long way towards reminding you and your partner of your connection.

As the weeks pass, however, and life returns to normal—or at least, to a new version of normal—you may be surprised to find that your sexual self is not just a memory from the past. And as long as you get the go-ahead from your healthcare provider, you can begin to resume your sexual relationship at a pace that's right for you. While some women find that they're eager to jump back into things, others may have some concerns . . .

- **Will intercourse hurt?** The answer is maybe. While some women are able to resume having intercourse without any problem, others may have some discomfort or pain, particularly if they've had an episiotomy or stitches for a perineum or vaginal tear. Some women have found that short-term use of a vaginal dilator helpful, while others have benefitted from perineum massage and/or regular Kegel exercises. In any case, be aware that your vagina, uterus, and cervix are still healing, and are likely to be sensitive to the thrusting of the penis during intercourse, so ask your partner to be extra gentle. Generally speaking, any physical discomfort during intercourse should improve over time; if difficulties persist, a healthcare provider should be consulted.
- **Will I still be able to have an orgasm?** Yes. During vaginal childbirth, the baby emerges from the vagina. Since the source of a woman's orgasm is her clitoris, and not her vagina, there is no reason for orgasm to be affected.
- **Is my vagina permanently changed after vaginal delivery?** Not structurally, unless affected by unexpected medical complications. Still, it may feel "looser" (if you gave birth to a large baby) or tighter (if you had a snug episiotomy repair). In the case of an uneventful vaginal delivery, it is perfectly normal for the vagina to feel somewhat looser following birth, and will restore itself to its prior state within three months or so.
- **I gave birth vaginally and can't seem to control when I pee!** Though few like to discuss it, and many are reluctant to bring it up with their healthcare provider, urinary (and fecal) incontinence are often a fact of the postpartum period, the result of fatigued

muscles, a contracting uterus, or other medical reasons. While it may be uncomfortable (and embarrassing!), it is quite common and usually reverses itself within approximately six to twelve months. In the meantime, we recommend emptying your bladder regularly and keeping a sense of humor.

- **What if I had a C-section?** In the case of caesarean birth, there may be tenderness at the surgical site as well as in the uterus; generally speaking, however, the vagina is not affected, posing fewer direct concerns when it comes to resuming sexual activity.

- **Will I ever feel sexy again?** While it's hard to imagine ever feeling sexual with spit-up on your clothes and milk leaking from your breasts, in the vast majority of cases, just as your body will return to its pre-pregnancy state, so will your sexual interest. When it comes to sex after childbirth, as always, we like to remind our patients that a woman's most significant sexual organ is her mind. So be patient with yourself, and ask your partner for patience as well. While you cannot jump into intercourse until you get the go-ahead from your healthcare provider, typically around the six weeks mark, in the meantime, there is no reason you can't enjoy other forms of affection and sexual contact, if you so desire.

———

Facing Postpartum Depression

If you have struggled with depression or anxiety before and/or during pregnancy, you are more susceptible to developing postpartum depression following childbirth. Postpartum depression, also known as PPD, can manifest in any number of ways, from feelings of sadness, hopelessness, anger, and helplessness to feelings of guilt and inadequacy. When it comes to postpartum depression, it's worth keeping in mind that we cannot separate our bodies from our minds, meaning that it can also show up in physical symptoms, like decreased appetite or an inability to sleep.

While there is a strong physiological component to PPD, our life circumstances also play a significant role in determining whether we are at risk. Women who are in an unhappy or dysfunctional relationships are at particular risk for experiencing PPD, as are new mothers who lack adequate social and family resources. In other words, cultivating some kind of supportive network around you as you recover from birth and get used to motherhood is critical. If you don't have a partner you can count on to share some of the burden, do your best to seek support elsewhere, such as a new moms' support network, which are plentiful online. Getting adequate rest and nutrition are also critical in keeping our bodies and minds healthy, as is moderate exercise (even a fifteen-minute walk outside can go a long way towards lifting one's spirits).

While feeling sad or overwhelmed is completely normal during the postpartum period, it is vital that we pay attention to depression symptoms, including anger, neglecting the baby, and fear of hurting the baby, that do not go away or get better with time. So if you have been experiencing any of the above for more than a couple weeks, it is worth a visit to your healthcare provider to help you assess the situation and make a plan towards recovery, which will typically include medication and/or psychotherapy.

Miscarriage: Confronting Your Loss

Despite the fact that miscarriage - spontaneous loss of pregnancy before the 20th week, usually a result of a genetic or health problem - is a fairly common experience for women, it still remains unclear why some pregnancies follow through to term and others spontaneously terminate. And the fact that it is common certainly does nothing to ease the disappointment and sense of loss if you are the one going through it.

Unlike pregnancy, the loss of a pregnancy is typically a very private experience. Because most women who miscarry do so within the early weeks of the first trimester, often before others even know they're pregnant, many women end up dealing with the loss on their own. If friends and family are already aware of the pregnancy, it can be painful to tell them relatively soon after having delivered the happy news.

Every woman responds to her miscarriage differently. Some women seem to take it in stride, seeing it as their bodies' way of letting them know that something wasn't right with the pregnancy, while others fall into deep mourning, even if they were only pregnant a few weeks.

For example, one of our patients, who had endured eight miscarriages, told us that she had come to see them as "mother nature trying to tell me something." After her final miscarriage, she and her husband decided to adopt and now have two happy, healthy children. Another one of our patients, however, became so distraught when she miscarried at six weeks that her loss began to consume her life; she named her unborn fetus and talked about him incessantly, joined multiple support groups, and was unable to be intimate with her husband for over a year. Eventually, she was convinced to see a psychotherapist and was prescribed anti-depressants to help her cope with her emotional pain.

For those who are suffering, the pain is often made worse because it is a difficult subject to talk about (and there are no public rituals to help you mourn your loss). Meanwhile, well-intentioned friends and family members can often be insensitive when trying to offer words of comfort. Comments like "It was meant to be," "It's God's way," or, if you already have a child, "At least you have one," are unlikely to make you feel any better and may even make you feel worse. If feelings of sadness and despair persist, it may be worth exploring counseling to help you cope with your loss. (If you experience multiple miscarriages, you may be considered high-risk and will require more watchful medical care, which may include genetic counseling and fertility testing; you may also benefit from psychotherapy or, in some cases, relationship counseling to help you—and your partner—manage the feelings of helplessness and frustration that often arise.)

When it comes to "moving on" from the experience and trying to get pregnant again, there are no hard and fast rules. Each woman must decide for herself if and when she is ready to try again. If the miscarriage occurred during the early part of the first trimester, the chances for conceiving again within a relatively short period of time are high. If the miscarriage took place later in the pregnancy, it is still very possible to get pregnant again, though it may take more time, as your body recovers and renews a regular menstrual and ovulation cycle. Once again, every woman's body will recover differently, so as long as you have medical clearance, our advice is to keep trying. The good news is that most women who experience miscarriage go on to have full-term pregnancies and healthy babies.

Choosing to Terminate

Whether you are single or married, in your teens or in your forties, opting to end a pregnancy is never an easy decision. The elective termination of a pregnancy takes a physiological, hormonal, and emotional toll on the body and mind regardless of the reason behind it, and is often accompanied by feelings of shame, guilt, and depression. One need not place a moral judgment on the choice to acknowledge the impact that an abortion may have on a woman's life, in some cases lasting years after the medical procedure has taken place. In our work with patients, we have found that while emotional support before the procedure is part of the process, counseling afterwards is not, despite it being vital to emerging from the experience unscathed. When seeking counseling, look for a therapist who is nonjudgmental, and do ask her about her own views regarding termination - you want to find the right person to hold your hand through the journey of healing.

The Challenge Of Infertility

Wanting to become a parent while struggling to get (or stay) pregnant can be one of the loneliest, most challenging experiences that a woman—or a couple—will face. In some cases, a healthcare provider or fertility specialist will be able to identify the cause, and whether it originates in the man (such as low sperm count or limited sperm mobility) or in the woman (such as endometriosis or various ovulation problems). But while there are plenty of possible causes—including everything from workplace toxins to advanced maternal age to a history of cancer treatment—why conception seems to happen so effortlessly for some couples and poses so much pain and frustration for others is something that is not fully understood by modern medicine.

It's worth bearing in mind that each woman's struggle with infertility is unique: some of us are unable to get pregnant at all, while others may be dealing with multiple miscarriages or pregnancies that are otherwise unviable, as in the case of an ectopic pregnancy. Some of us will remain committed to the notion that we "should" be able to conceive naturally, while others will take advantage of assisted reproduction technology at the earliest opportunity. For some women, the journey through infertility will end with children, whether through assisted pregnancy or adoption, while others may choose to make peace with life without children.

Infertility can affect women of any age, culture, sexual orientation, marital status, education, or income bracket. One woman we know in her mid-twenties, whom we'll call Yvonne, had been struggling to get pregnant with her husband for years. The fact that she was "only" twenty-six made her feel even more isolated and alone.

"I feel like a total failure," she told us bluntly. "And what's worse is that people are always asking us, 'When are you going to have a baby already? What are you waiting for?' So many of our friends already have babies, and some are already pregnant with their second. It's gotten to the point where I find myself making up reasons to avoid seeing them."

Tanya, another woman we know, who, at age 41, has been undergoing fertility treatments since getting married in her late thirties, has written openly on her personal blog about the extent of her exhaustion with the whole process. "I am at the end of my rope—emotionally, physically, and financially. I'm starting to wonder if all of this is really worth it, but my husband and I still can't escape the sense that without a child, there's something missing in our lives."

With infertility taking a physical, hormonal, and emotional toll, there's no question that it will affect your sexual relationship as well. This is understandable given that all of a sudden, sex can begin to feel like work—and not just any work, but high-pressure work, with the highest of stakes. Not to mention the fact that doing it "on demand," according to your ovulation cycle, does not feel particularly intimate or erotic—especially if you know you'll be reporting the results to your medical fertility team. While some couples will be able to withstand these pressures—in fact, we have seen some relationships emerge stronger—other couples find that the stresses caused by infertility end up being more than their relationship can bear. Not surprisingly, it is often the woman who experiences these stresses most acutely. As Tanya shared with us, her depression has begun to have a corrosive effect on her marriage. "I still love my husband," Tanya reported, "But at this point, I've just lost any interest in being intimate with him. I can no longer even think about sex without thinking about the baby I wish we had."

Indeed, in addition to experiencing a sense of loss or helplessness, feelings of jealousy are also perfectly natural—and very common. Unfortunately, that does not typically make such feelings any easier to manage if you are the one experiencing them. For this reason, it's imperative that in addition to any reproductive assistance, you also seek psychological or other therapeutic help—ideally, with a therapist who has experience in the field of infertility—which is vital to working through the range of painful emotions that inevitably arise throughout the process.

When to Get Help

Generally speaking, a couple is thought to be struggling with infertility after nine to twelve months of trying to conceive naturally. If this describes your experience, the first thing to remember is that you are not alone. The second thing to keep in mind is that medical help is available, with fertility treatments advancing every day. While there remains a wide range of success rates, the most common treatments include one or more of the following:

- *In Vitro Fertilization (IVF)*—utilizing your own eggs or donor eggs.
- *Intrauterine Insemination (IUI)*, also known as artificial insemination—utilizing your partner's sperm or donor sperm.
- *Clomid (Clomiphene citrate)*—a drug intended to stimulate ovulation in women and/or increase sperm count in men.
- *Surrogacy*—engaging another woman to carry the fetus to term, using either your eggs (in which case the surrogate may be known as a gestational carrier) or her own.

Because the physiological—and financial—costs of fertility treatments can be enormous, we encourage our patients to maintain as much perspective as possible in the journey towards parenthood. For many couples, exploring adoption is a wonderful option. No matter which route one chooses, it is worth keeping in mind that while assisted reproduction technologies may help some of us, many women have gone on to lead full and productive lives with—or without—biological children of their own.

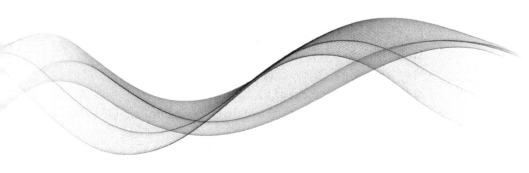

Chapter Three

The Myth of Perfect Sex

Am I doing it Wrong?

"**A**m I doing it wrong?" This is one of the most common questions we hear in our office, along with the related questions: "*Are we doing it wrong?*" "*What am I missing?*" and "*Does everyone else know something about sex that I don't?*" In our quest for sexual pleasure, excitement, and fulfillment, it's totally understandable that at one point or another we may find ourselves wondering about what it is exactly that other people are doing in bed.

There's nothing wrong with maintaining a healthy curiosity about human sexuality. And some of us may be able to learn a great deal by having frank and open discussions with our sisters or closest friends. In fact, lifting the taboo against talking about sex has helped many of us become more sexually comfortable with our partners and ourselves. A problem arises only when we begin comparing ourselves to other women and use their experiences—real or imagined—as a basis for judging our own. This is especially so when we use the media as a guideline for what we "should" look like and how it "should" feel and the kind of sex we "should" be having. And because we're bombarded with these "shoulds" almost everywhere we turn, it's no wonder that so many us end up feeling inadequate in some way:

- I'm too fat/too skinny to feel sexy.
- My breasts are too small/too big.
- My partner's too fat/too skinny.
- My partner's not as sexy as the men I see on TV.
- We never do it on the kitchen table/up against the wall like they do in the movies.
- My boyfriend expects me to wear kinky lingerie like women in the Victoria's Secret catalog.
- My partner wants to do it in a position he saw in the movies, but it's uncomfortable for me.
- Do other couples have more fun than we do?
- Is sex really supposed to be two hours long?
- Why don't I orgasm from intercourse?

Too many of us have been led to believe that everyone else is having all the fun. We think that because we see it in the movies, it must be real. We think that because we read about it online, everybody must be doing it. We think that because we read about it in magazines, it must be good. Whether we're struggling not to compare our sex lives with those we read about, or living with a partner whose understanding of sex is based exclusively on what he sees onscreen, it can be difficult to sort out what we want from what we've been told to want, especially if our partners are pressuring us to "live up to" a sexual fantasy. As one of our patients told us, "For some reason, my husband thinks that having a good sex life means that intercourse should last for hours. It gets to the point where I often have to stop and ask him, 'are you done yet?' and he says, 'no, I'm still doing it, like in the movies.' I don't want to hurt his feelings, but I don't really find anything enjoyable about marathon-style sex. My vagina can't take it, and neither can my psyche."

Not long ago, another patient of ours, whom we'll call Cynthia, told us, "I have a low sex drive; it is something I've always known about myself. I was never into being sexual several times per week, unlike my sister and my friends. For years I've been blaming it on other causes, such as having kids, occasional yeast infections, etc., but if I take away all these excuses, the truth is there: twenty years into my marriage, and I am not like the others. What IS wrong with me?"

There seemed to be no doubt in Cynthia's mind that she was suffering from some kind of sexual dysfunction. Yet when we asked her if the sexual experiences she did have were satisfying, she immediately replied that they were. When we inquired about her husband's feelings on the subject, she explained that he had slowed down sexually over the years, but had no complaints whatsoever about their sexual encounters.

When we let Cynthia know that we saw no problem, given that they were both content, she insisted that she and her husband "must be missing out on something." After all, she pointed out, "Other people seem to be doing it a lot more often than we do, and the media is full of advice about how to increase libido. I wish my sex drive were stronger, but at the same time, all the pressure puts me out of my comfort zone."

We reassured her that everyone has his or her own individual sexual template, and that each relationship has its own sexual style. While we suggested that she and her husband might consider expanding their sexual repertoire by trying new things and/or work on enhancing their intimate zone (see Chapter Five), we explained that it was unlikely she would be able to alter her sex drive per se, which, for women, is subject to life's cycles, hormonal changes, state of mind, and the typical diminishing of sexual interest over the course of a long-term relationship.

"I didn't realize how quickly I blamed myself for being 'faulty,'" Cynthia said, "and how much my thinking and expectations were affected by the sex messages from the media. Now I wonder what really goes on behind others' closed doors . . ."

The First Time

For some of us, our first intercourse may have been a positive experience. But for many of us, it was more likely to have been awkward or uncomfortable, if not downright painful. We may have felt scared, excited, ashamed, confused, relieved—or we may have not known what we were feeling at all. Whether we were in our teens or well into adulthood, whether it was a casual encounter or on our wedding night, the actual experience of "losing our virginity" probably did not match the romantic image we had in our heads. In reality, for the vast majority of women, the "first time" tends to be more of a learning experience than a magical moment. The truth is that for most of us, learning how to enjoy intercourse is just that—a learning process, which takes time, practice, and patience. And yet, based on what we see on television and in the movies, "losing it" is an unforgettable, life-changing awesome event, the singular moment when a girl becomes a woman.

Unfortunately, this myth is perpetuated not only by the mainstream media, but by the religious media as well. Those of us who were raised in religious communities were not only unlikely to have had previous sexual experiences to prepare for a mature sexual relationship, but we were also likely taught that the first intercourse is reserved for marriage, a moment not only of great intimacy with one's spouse, but a moment of great spiritual significance as well. So if it does not go according to plan—whether it is physically impossible (see Chapter Nine), unbearably painful (again, see Chapter Eight), or otherwise emotionally traumatic—we may feel that we have failed, not only physically, but spiritually. Talk about pressure!

No matter what one's religious or cultural background, we encourage young women to educate themselves about their sexuality, and the mechanics of intercourse, as much as possible. As always, knowledge is power, and power means preparation. Knowing about the importance of foreplay, lubrication, and most importantly, communication with one's partner about what's comfortable and what's not, are vital first steps in ensuring that the first time is memorable for the right reasons.

Sex and the Media

Just look around and you'll notice how consistently the media trots out the same clichés about heterosexual sex, over and over again. For one thing, the couple is always "into it," forever moving smoothly about their sexual actions, knowing exactly what they like and how they like it, all body parts fitting just so. The woman is *always* interested/eager/ready for the man, and both experience an instant, mind-blowing simultaneous orgasm without any effort at all. Not to mention the fact that there is typically only one model for what a sexually desirable woman looks like, which ignores the wide variety of real women's bodies.

Indeed, the media continuously bombard us with the message that "If you look like [fill in the blank with the name of the current "hot" actor or actress], you'll have a good sex life." And it's not just movies and TV—popular athletes are also representatives of the media; it's no coincidence that they are also encouraged to look "sexy" to increase viewership. After all, how many people would tune in to watch women's beach volleyball without the bikinis? It's also not a coincidence that the most attractive athletes are paid big bucks to endorse everything from watches to breakfast cereal. In fact, advertising, in its many forms, tells us, "If you buy [fill in the blank with the latest gadget or luxury item], you'll have a good sex life." It's certainly no secret that sexual images are used to sell everything from cars to perfume to movies to beer to cosmetics to clothes, to sexual aids . . . you get the idea. Whether we like it or not, the reality is that the media establishes the standards, role models, and formulas for what sex ought to look like and what we ought to look like while having it. It is in the business of marketing an idealized vision of sex and sexuality.

Because of the all-encompassing presence of the media in our lives, we begin consuming images of idealized sexual fantasy when we are still very young and highly suggestible. They bury themselves in our psyches, and over the course of our development play a key role in determining our sexual templates. Our training, in other words, in what constitutes "perfect sex" starts early and goes deep, *whether or not we are consciously aware of it*, so that by the time we reach our teenage years and begin to actively explore our sexuality, we already have specific expectations of both ourselves and others.

It is worth noting that because sexuality is not openly discussed—or discussed at all—in many families, cultures, and traditions, the ever-present media is, for many people, their only avenue for learning about it. This is a particularly cruel reality given the fact that sex in the media is orchestrated, sensationalized sex designed for maximum titillation; it does not reflect the reality of how individuals actually experience sex for themselves. While there's no doubt this causes unspoken anxieties for both sexes, it can be particularly difficult for women, who are more likely than men to measure their self-esteem according to conventional, media-driven images of beauty, fitness, and sexual attractiveness. At times, even the medical community takes its cues from the media as a guide for what's considered "normal."

Not only does the media not take into account sexual individuality, it does not make room for the natural process of aging or the inevitable cycles of life. In the movies, on television, and online, characters exist in a parallel universe of eternal youth, in which individuals over a certain age are regarded as sexually undesirable. Once again, it is women who are disproportionally affected, given that male actors are often considered "sexy" or "distinguished" well into their seventies and even eighties, while female actors are—with rare exceptions—relegated to playing asexual matriarchs. While the disparity between how women and men are depicted as they get older continues onscreen, in real life, it is further complicated by the surging popularity of drugs like Viagra or Cialis, designed to enhance male sexual performance and function, further extending the media-driven image of eternal male virility. The result? Older women, much as they may still crave intimacy, are compelled to engage in and perform sexually beyond the scope of what is comfortable for them.

It's not only images of sexual "perfection" that have the potential to embed themselves in our psyches. Some of our patients report having been so deeply affected by behaviors and items they saw in the movies or on television that it had a long-lasting impact on their sexual choices. There is much reason to be wary of the influence the media has on our daily perspective of women and sexuality

Surgery and the Quest for Perfection

In recent years, the pursuit of sexual perfection has taken on new proportions (and profits) as increasing numbers of men and women are opting to undergo voluntary surgical procedures (ouch!) in the hopes of looking "young and sexy" forever. Following in the footsteps of other forms of elective cosmetic surgery, the business of genital rejuvenation has grown into a multi-billion dollar industry. Indeed, there's no question that sex sells!

Today, there are countless surgical options available—and heavily marketed—to women, ranging from breast augmentation and surgical vaginal tightening to labiaplasty (to reduce the size of the labial folds) and hymenoplasty (to restore the hymen). But women aren't the only ones who face cultural, and sometimes personal, pressures to undergo these "enhancements." While women receive the subtle, and not-so-subtle, message that the "virginal" vagina is the apex of desirable femininity, men are no less burdened by cultural dictates to be "real men"—strong, virile, and expert sexual performers. Towards that end, it is no wonder that procedures like girth enhancement (penile widening) and phalloplasty (penile lengthening), not to mention inflatable penile implants, are becoming increasingly common.

Premised on an ever-elusive goal of virginity (for women) and virility (for men), is it any wonder that individuals who choose to undergo these surgeries often remain plagued by underlying insecurities and relationship difficulties even after the surgical wounds have healed?

One of our patients, a woman in her late twenties whom we'll call Andrea, arrived at our office saying there was "something very wrong with me." As we spoke with her, we learned that she had recently undergone a labiaectomy, a surgical procedure to shorten the labia minora (the inner lips of the vulva), which she claimed were "too long." Andrea's procedure had been performed by a top gynecological surgeon, and cosmetically speaking, the surgery had been an unqualified success. Yet Andrea insisted that she was still unhappy with the shape of her vulva, convinced that it was the source of a recent break-up. Upon examination and further discussion, we discovered that Andrea had opted for the surgery in a last-ditch attempt to save her relationship with her boyfriend, who she knew had been cheating on her. In her mind, she explained, having the surgery would make her boyfriend want her, not someone else.

Because we sensed that Andrea's distress had less to do with the size of her inner lips and more to do with her internal turmoil, we referred her to a trusted psychotherapist. Ultimately, it took quite a bit of counseling to help Andrea realize that what she needed to get her life back on track was an emotional intervention, not a surgical one.

Another one of our patients, a woman in her mid-thirties named Kristin, was shocked when, following the birth of their third child, her husband promptly told her that he was not happy with her "down there." "I want you to be nice and tight," he informed her. Feeling defeated, and desperately wanting to keep her husband from seeking sexual satisfaction outside their marriage, she made an appointment with a plastic surgeon to discuss undergoing vaginoplasty. To Kristin's dismay, however, the doctor said he was unwilling to recommend the surgery for her, given that her vagina was absolutely normal. Sadly, Kristin's husband left her several months later, prompting her to regret not seeking out another surgeon who would have been willing to perform the surgery. Once again, it took months of therapy for Kristin to realize that the so-called "problem" with her vagina was never a problem at all, and that there was no surgery in the world that would have prevented her husband from leaving.

Porn and Relationships

Pornography, or porn, as it is more commonly known, is nothing new. The portrayal of women and men—but most typically women—in sexually suggestive images, or engaged explicitly in sexual acts, has been around since ancient times. For centuries, pornography was available in the form of wall carvings and paintings, statues and figurines, erotic books, magazines, photographs, postcards, and beginning in the late nineteenth century, movies. But as most of us know, with the invention of the Internet, the availability of porn has—almost quite literally—exploded, and is now more readily available than ever before. And with porn so accessible—at the touch of a button and in the comfort of one's own space, wherever that is—it has lured increasing numbers of consumers.

Geared almost exclusively towards a male audience, porn tends to depict sexual acts in the most physical, sensationalistic way possible—removing any emotional or relational aspects from the equation. More often than not, porn films are populated by female actresses who conform to an idealized (and often surgically or digitally enhanced) image of what women "should" look like. Furthermore, these actresses—who are, as many viewers forget, *acting*—are ready to engage in penetration or perform oral sex immediately and to do so for hours on end. Of course, it bears mentioning that the male porn actors are no less idealized—with muscular physiques, large penises, and erections that seem to last forever.

There is no question that porn's increased accessibility is placing increased pressure on many relationships. Not only can excessive porn consumption lead to unrealistic expectations for where, when, and how couples engage sexually, it can place particular pressure on women (often via their partners) to look and behave in ways that may not feel authentic or comfortable. In one case, a married mother of two young children came to see us for sexual counseling because her husband had become increasingly obsessed with Internet porn, in particular a site specializing in large-breasted women. "He seemed to like my body just fine before he got into porn," she told us, "but now he's insisting that I undergo breast enlargement so I can look more like them." In another instance, we were contacted by a woman in her mid-fifties who had noticed her partner's declining interest in sex before discovering that he was seeking his sexual satisfaction in porn. "Now, whenever we do have sex," she explained, "he criticizes our experience, or worse, uses a rating system to evaluate his sexual performance."

Another problem is that as a result of porn's ubiquity, it can be nearly impossible for some viewers to control their habits. And like any other addiction, its excessive consumption may lead to evasive behavior, financial ruin, and relationship crises. As one woman recently told us, "I keep catching my partner shutting off his computer as soon as I walk into the room. I'm pretty sure it's because he's watching porn, which I'm not thrilled about, but what bothers me more is how secretive he's become."

When Porn Becomes an Addiction

In more extreme cases, porn addiction can be a slippery slope that leads an individual down a path of emotional and, in some instances, financial ruin, as happened to a patient's husband who became so obsessed with getting his pornography fix that he began calling in sick to work, which eventually led to losing his job, and not long after, his marriage. In other cases, individuals may go into debt visiting online sites that require pay-to-view membership fees. Like any other addiction, porn addiction is a symptom of deep underlying dysfunction and/or inability to deal with life stressors. It is important to bring awareness of it into public consciousness so that affected individuals, as well as their partners, can receive the treatment and support they need.

Of course, a partner's preoccupation with porn—even if it has not developed into a full-fledged addiction—may lead a woman to feel insecure about her relationship in any number of ways:

- I'm not a porn star! I feel like my boyfriend expects me to act like one.
- Why does my partner have to watch pornography before he can have sex with me?
- I feel like I'm competing with the Internet.
- Is my husband cheating on me? Isn't it adultery?
- He doesn't need me anymore.
- How could he do this? Doesn't he have any respect for me?
- It's against our religion.

And yet . . . that does not mean that porn is necessarily always bad for relationships—as long as couples are willing to communicate honestly. "I always thought that the fact that my husband watched porn meant that I wasn't enough for him," a patient of ours in her early thirties named Jenny once confided. "It used to really bother me. Then, one day, I decided that instead of allowing myself to feel hurt and angry, that I would ask him about it, in the most non-judgmental way I could. Obviously, it was not an easy subject to bring up, but I'm so glad I did. We ended up having one of the most honest conversations we've ever had. My husband explained that for him, porn was a once-in-a-while stress reliever, something that let him shut out all of his stresses and go into a world of complete fantasy. He assured me that it in no way took away from his attraction to me. In fact, he said that after watching porn, he often felt more attracted to me, not less."

Jenny described the conversation as a real turning point for her and her husband, who both began to talk more openly with each other about their sexual fantasies, which Jenny said she had previously felt too embarrassed and ashamed to share. They even began experimenting with watching porn together. "I was surprised to find that watching porn with my husband could actually really turn me on," Jenny told us. "That is something I never would have expected." But the most important revelation, she said, was learning that she and her husband did not have to hide anything from each other. "I learned that there was room in our relationship to talk about things I had always thought were too private to talk about with anyone—even my husband."

Indeed, our clinical experience has shown that porn—as well as other media portrayals of sex—can, in some cases, be used as tools to help couples enhance their sexual connection. As long as we do not take it as "gospel," or obsessively compare ourselves with the images depicted onscreen, porn can serve as a springboard for helping us to identify what turns us on and what doesn't. Once we are able to respect ourselves and our bodies—and that of our partner, if we have one—there is no reason why we can't allow porn to serve as a guide for bringing more creativity to our sexual repertoires and helping us to expand our "sexual menus" (see Chapter Four).

For women who are interested in further exploring the world of porn, either with or without a partner, keep in mind that much of mainstream pornography is geared towards the male sexual template, and may strike you as boring, mechanical, unimaginative, or downright offensive, so take the time to do your research. Today, there is a wide range of erotica available, both in hard copy and online, some of it geared specifically toward the female psyche, depicting not just body parts in action but also a storyline with romance, affection, and feelings. Of course, not all of us will feel comfortable using media-generated images to inspire our own sexual imaginations, whether for religious or other personal reasons. It is important to know that if we choose to refrain, that is an acceptable choice as well.

Does Watching Porn Mean He's Cheating on Me?

"My husband watches porn every night when he comes home from work." "My boyfriend seems to spend more and more time on the Internet—with the door locked." "I was borrowing my partner's computer one day and was shocked to see the history of sites he's been visiting." These are just a few of the comments we hear from our patients, often followed by the question, "Is he cheating on me?"

Faced with feelings ranging from confusion to betrayal, some women will choose not to raise the subject with their partners, preferring to deal with their feelings on their own, or in some cases, allowing them to fester. Other women will opt to confront their partners, only to be met with typical responses such as, "How can you accuse me of cheating on you? I'm not doing anything wrong," or "I never met her in person," or "I never touched her body, so why do you get offended?"

Indeed, the use of pornography raises the larger question of how we define infidelity. In some cases, porn can open the door to real-life infidelity. But in other cases, even if one's partner is not physically engaging in sexual activity with another person, it may still feel like infidelity. It is important to remember that both forms of infidelity—virtual or actual—can be equally hurtful, not to mention harmful to the relationship and to a woman's sense of self. Given the differences between male and female sexual templates (see Chapter Six), and because a woman's sexuality is filtered through her mind and emotions whereas a man's sexuality is largely focused on the realm of the physical, their opinions about what constitutes unfaithful behavior may differ.

Nevertheless, that is only a starting place. As always, communication is vital: discuss your questions, fears, sense of betrayal, and concerns with your partner in a candid way. Rather than engage in the blame-and-shame game, allow your partner the opportunity to present his own feelings on the subject. For some couples, seeking the help of a licensed psychotherapist or sexual counselor may be necessary to sort out the crisis, discuss available solutions, and offer support and guidance, whether you decide to move forward in the relationship or end it.

Embracing Reality

So what do we do with all the images of sensationalized sex that permeate our daily lives? How can we distance ourselves from the manufactured sexuality that pops up every time we surf the Internet or turn on the television? Is it possible to create a realistic sexual model?

An important first step is learning how to embrace ourselves, in all our individuality. We each vary in our looks, in our sexual wants and needs, and in our sexual expectations. Furthermore, we all change as we move through relationships, and stages of life: we bring our sexual history to each new relationship, and explore the unique sexual chemistry that will vary with each new partner. We may find, for example, that we're more sexually assertive in one relationship, and more passive in another. Or we may find within a long-term relationship that our desires change over time. As we grow and change as human beings, so does our sexuality.

If you constantly compare yourself to images in the media, or if you find yourself judging your sex life based on what you see in the movies, it might help to open up a dialogue on the subject with your partner. You may be surprised to discover that he has been grappling with his own feelings, questions, or self-doubt. If you are single, discuss with a trusted friend or a counselor. Another idea is to make a list of the ways in which you feel dissatisfied with your sex life, as well as a list of things you want your sex life to include moving forward, and share it with your partner. Or you might consider showing him or her this chapter to get the conversation going. For those of us dealing with particularly difficult sexual or relationship challenges, counseling may be necessary. But for some, the antidote to the onslaught of cultural messages may be as simple as choosing to educate ourselves about sex and sexuality. Time and time again, we have found that sexual education is the key to leaving the media behind and bringing a healthy dose of reality to the bedroom.

We hope it goes without saying that this does not mean there's no room for fantasy! Nobody wants their sex lives to get stale—we want our sexual encounters to be fun, joyous, and full of exploration. As we've discussed, our fantasies, as well as our partners' fantasies, can inspire us to get more in touch with ourselves as sexual beings. The key is making sure that our fantasies feel comfortable and blend realistically with who we are—and that they don't violate our core sense of dignity. So allow yourself to enjoy a sense of play, either by yourself or with your partner.

It's all too easy to become convinced that the definition of "perfect sex" comes from without—when the reality is that is can only come from within. So . . . what makes for perfect sex?

- When it's safe and consensual.
- When you feel happy and satisfied.
- When you feel comfortable, both physically and emotionally.
- When you feel free to voice your desires, opinions, and concerns.
- When you feel your partner cares about your experience.
- When you are able to both give and receive.
- When there is room to experiment and explore.
- When you can be you!

It is precisely because sexuality is such an individual experience that we do not (and, for that matter, cannot) claim to have all the answers. Rather, our goal is to offer reassurance to every woman reading this book to give yourself permission to follow your natural instincts—if it feels good for you, it is good. Perfect sex is not about what you see in the media—it's about paying attention to **your** wants and needs to find the sex that is perfect for you.

Where Are The Condoms?

Among the many myths that the media perpetrates about sex, one of the most dangerous is that condoms aren't necessary when it comes to new relationships, let alone one-time sexual encounters. When the leading lady and leading man lock eyes on the big screen, there is often limited verbal foreplay, never mind a frank conversation about sexual history, let alone an acknowledgment that one or both of them is carrying a Sexually Transmitted infection (STI). According to Hollywood, the young and sexy are simply invulnerable to contracting any of the innumerable infections that are so easily transmitted through unprotected vaginal, anal, and/or oral sex, including HPV, genital herpes, chlamydia, gonorrhea, and HIV, to name just a few. With the media serving as so many people's model for how sex should proceed, it probably shouldn't come as a surprise that a large number of our patients report a reluctance to use condoms in their sexual encounters. At first, we thought it was because they were not aware of the risks, until we realized that was not the case. Rather, the reasons they cited tended to be more in line with wanting to fulfill an idealized sexual fantasy . . .

▶ "It will affect the spontaneity of our sex."
▶ "But he is a clean, good, responsible guy!"
▶ "He gets an annual physical exam by his doctor."
▶ "He was only with two other women before me . . ."
▶ "I am uncomfortable talking to him about using condoms."
▶ "He says he doesn't like to use condoms."
▶ "But intercourse is not as good for him if he is wearing a condom."
▶ "I don't want to lose him by insisting on it."
▶ "He says he is okay and I want to believe him."
▶ "I never knew that oral herpes could be transmitted to the genitals."
▶ "Should I talk to him about STIs? Is it really that important?"
▶ "But they don't use condoms in the movies!"

And so we continue to treat women who have contracted STIs from unprotected sex. It is worth remembering that **there is no way to be 100% sure if your partner is a carrier for an STI**. Even if he claims to have just been tested, to have a clean bill of health, and to visit his healthcare provider regularly, few people realize that sexually transmitted infections can lie dormant for months before showing up. The only way to ensure you are both free of STIs is to repeat sexual testing one year into your monogamous relationship. Despite what the media may tell us, sexually transmitted infections are very real—and in some cases very dangerous—consequences of not taking ownership of our sexual health.

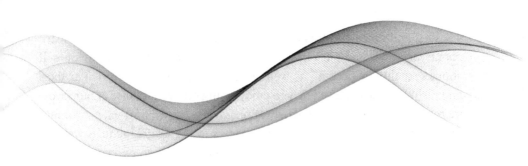

Chapter Four

The Sexual Menu

Exploring Your Options

What do you think of when you hear the word "sex"? For many people, those three letters conjure up only one thing: intercourse, or to be more specific, penetrative heterosexual vaginal intercourse. Indeed, in mainstream culture, this is the activity that determines the presence or absence of virginity, and that, across religious traditions, constitutes the definitive marital act. Even today's pop culture, as evidenced in movies, music videos, and television, celebrates penis-vagina coitus as the ultimate goal—or even the "prize"—of any romantic situation.

From our perspective, this is a limited and outdated view of human sexuality, which does not begin to describe the myriad possibilities for intimate contact with another person, let alone with ourselves. In reality, sex is about so much more than the act of coitus. While it can take on a variety of forms, which we refer to in this chapter and throughout the book as the "*Sexual Menu*," sexual activity is not just about what body part goes where; it encompasses any thought, activity, or practice that pertains to arousal and to erotic feelings. Rather than rely on the glorified images of missionary-style sex peddled by the media, we encourage each and every woman to define sex for herself.

First and foremost, this means cultivating the self-confidence to learn about your own body. It also means taking the time to educate yourself about sexuality in general, as well as to explore your own particular likes and dislikes. Just as we're likely to enjoy trying different dishes at our favorite restaurant depending on what we're craving, it's vital for us, as women, to know that we have options when it comes to the sexual menu as well. So if you find that you and your partner have fallen into a rut, or if you find that your sexual relationship is defined primarily by your own boredom or disinterest, we encourage you to mix and match items on the menu and to not be afraid of trying something outside your comfort zone.

Like any skill worth acquiring, learning how to navigate our sexuality takes practice; our clinical experience has shown the time and energy spent doing so is well worth it, paying back dividends throughout our lives. We believe that sexuality works from the inside out, which means that the better we know ourselves, the better our sexual experiences with a partner, should we choose to have one, will be. It's worth remembering that learning how to accept pleasure is a journey in and of itself—and one that we hope you will find is **worth** taking.

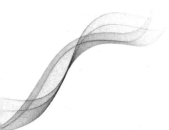

The Sexual Menu

(in no particular order)

- ▸ Masturbation
- ▸ Manual sex
- ▸ Dry sex

- ▸ Oral sex
- ▸ Anal sex
- ▸ Vaginal intercourse

The In's and Out's of Intercourse

Given that intercourse remains the default answer for what most people think of when they think about sex, and because it's an important feature of so many heterosexual relationships, it's a good place to begin a discussion of the sexual menu. While Merriam-Webster defines sexual intercourse as "sexual activity between two people; especially sexual activity in which a man puts his penis into the vagina of a woman," we all know that it entails a lot more than the act of penetration. Of course, there are the physical and logistical aspects to consider: How do both partners agree on a position? How long does intercourse last? What if your partner is aroused but you are not? What if it's uncomfortable or even painful? There are also a wide range of emotional and psychological factors that come into play: How do you feel about your partner in general? Are you truly in the mood to be intimate? Are you able to communicate your feelings and preferences, and is he open to hearing them?

Unfortunately, many men—and women!—still tend to think about intercourse from the male point of view. The physical realities of intercourse contribute to this perception, by simple virtue of the fact that a man must be aroused (i.e., erect) in order for intercourse to take place, while a woman, from a purely technical perspective, need not be. Even our understanding of what constitutes intercourse—the thrusting motion of the penis and the man's subsequent climax—remains very male-focused, a viewpoint that is, to a large extent, fostered by the medical community.

Indeed, the very focus on vaginal intercourse, often to the exclusion of other forms of sexual activity, betrays our culture's preoccupation with reproduction and with male sexual satisfaction. Because of all the emphasis on vaginal intercourse, many of us have never learned that **the act of penetration, in and of itself, does not equal female sexual arousal.** Although the penis is the primary male sexual organ, the vagina is *not* the primary female sexual organ, which remains one of the great misunderstandings about female sexuality. In truth, the female sexual organ is the clitoris, which can be found just north of the vagina. For this reason, the majority of women will not climax during intercourse unless direct or indirect clitoral stimulation is included as part of the activity. (For more on the clitoris and its role in achieving orgasm, see Chapter Five.)

For many of us, our feelings about intercourse may be complex and layered. Even if we are in healthy and nurturing relationships, we may find that we experience a wide spectrum of emotions about it, some of which we may not be able to articulate to ourselves, let alone to our partners. One of our patients, for example, explained her feelings this way: "Even though I love my husband very much, and I enjoy being sexually close to him, there is often something about having sex that makes me feel uneasy. It's hard for me to explain, but no matter how affectionate and loving he is, I still have this sense that he is the one 'doing something' to me while I am the one being 'done to'."

Our clinical experience has shown that this kind of response is not unusual, no matter how deeply we may try to bury it in our psyches. For this reason, we maintain that it is especially important for women to empower themselves during the act of vaginal intercourse, whether by choosing a sexual position that is pleasurable for them, opting to climax before, after, or simultaneously with their partner, guiding their partners' movements, or by any other means that helps them to remember that they are active and willing participants.

Finally, there is no rule that all sexual encounters must lead to intercourse! There is nothing wrong with you and your partner choosing to enjoy one or more items on the sexual menu without the assumption that things will inevitably conclude in penetrative sex. However, if and when you do choose to do so, read on for how to make sure the experience is as pleasurable as possible . . .

Choosing a position

While there are dozens—if not hundreds!—of possible positions for sexual intercourse, most couples will discover a few favorites that they return to again and again.

How do two people determine which positions work for them? Well, there are no rules, other than keeping an open mind and a flexible attitude. The main thing to remember is that finding what works best is not an exact science. For most of us, our favored sexual positions will evolve over the course of a relationship, or change depending on our chemistry with a new partner.

Finding positions that are comfortable and satisfying for both of you may require trying something you never thought you would, or encouraging your partner to try something that is new for him. While we generally encourage women to try new positions before they reject them, it is always within your rights to say "no" to something that feels physically painful or emotionally degrading. As the "hostess" to the penis, it's your prerogative to say which position—or positions—you prefer. While there are countless potential variations, the following is an overview of the most common sexual positions:

- Man on top, with the women lying beneath him, also known as "missionary style."
- Woman on top, with the man lying beneath her.
- Woman on her hands and knees, with the man behind her, also known as "doggy style."
- Woman and man lying side-by-side, also known as "spooning."
- Woman lying at the edge of the bed or reclining on a chair while the man enters her from a standing position.
- Both partners standing.

Keep in mind that taking the time to experiment with different positions is a worthwhile investment in learning about your sexual preferences, which may also shift and change depending on you or your partner's mood, the time of day, religious or cultural considerations, sexual orientation, erectile dysfunction issues, medical restrictions, use of sexual toys, what's happening in your relationship, etc. You may find that in some encounters, you enjoy the feeling of closeness that some couples experience during deep thrusting, which is typically best facilitated by the "missionary" position. Other times, you may crave the intimacy of intercourse minus the intensity of deep thrusting, in which case you and your partner might prefer to have intercourse "spooning" style, which allows for more minimal penile penetration.

Health, lifecycle events, and the natural process of aging also come into play. Milestones such as pregnancy and post-childbirth recovery may require adjustments to your repertoire. For example, some couples find woman-on-top, side-by-side, and "doggy style" to be the most comfortable positions during pregnancy, particularly in the later months. Finally, it's worth mentioning that the positions we enjoy in our twenties may simply no longer be realistic options as we get older. One of our patients in her mid-fifties, for example, had to explain to her husband after she'd undergone knee surgery that as much as they had once enjoyed it, she could simply no longer engage in "doggy style" sex. While communication and negotiation with your partner are vital components of any sexual encounter, remember that at the end of the day, the choice of whether, when, and how you are willing to engage is ultimately yours.

Making Modifications

In the movies, couples who decide to have intercourse magically fit together just so, but in real life, some of us may be facing medical issues that necessitate giving special attention to if, when, and how intercourse can take place. These considerations may include—but are not limited to—finding the right position that ensures maximum comfort for both of you; partial intercourse, in which the penis enters the vagina only partway; or in some instances, simulating intercourse with a sex accessory such as a dildo. Rather than focus on what the body can no longer do, we try to help our patients to see the possibilities that await them in customizing their sexual activity to fit their needs.

For example, if you or your partner suffers from multiple sclerosis, cerebral palsy, muscular dystrophy, or certain congenital conditions, adjustments will need to be made to ensure that intercourse is possible and comfortable for both of you. Similarly, if you or your partner are in the midst of, or recovering from cancer treatment, you may discover that you need to explore new ways of being intimate, particularly if you have undergone a surgical procedure for cervical, ovarian, or other gynecological cancers, which may affect the depth of the vagina. (See Chapter Ten for more on sexuality and cancer.) The same is true if a man suffers from Peyronie's disease, or has undergone intervention for prostate or testicular cancer.

Of course, in some situations, intercourse may be impossible altogether, but that doesn't mean that other items on the sexual menu can't be just as satisfying. If you are grappling with one of the above, or any other medical condition, remember that finding new avenues of sexual pleasure need not be a chore. For many individuals and couples, seeking the help of a licensed sex therapist can make all the difference in learning how to enjoy your new physique or that of your partner.

Just because intercourse by itself will not lead a woman to orgasm does not mean that your pleasure is not important! Patients often ask us how other couples "do it"—in other words, how do couples ensure that both the woman and the man end the encounter feeling satisfied? Our experience has shown that the most common answer is that they take turns. Often, the man will make sure his partner climaxes first, given that men typically enjoy prolonging their own state of arousal. Other couples will switch things around, with the man reaching climax first, followed by the woman. We recommend mixing it up and taking the time to experiment with different variations. Some women, for example, find intercourse more pleasurable after they've already climaxed, while others find their bodies are too sensitive for intercourse following orgasm.

Meanwhile, other couples engage in simultaneous stimulation, with the goal of timing their orgasms to coincide. For those who want to enjoy the pleasure of experiencing orgasm during intercourse, choose a position that offers your partner the easiest, most comfortable access to stimulate the clitoris. Alternatively, couples can practice synchronizing their rhythms during intercourse so that their levels of arousal grow in unison. This entails finding a comfortable position in which the man can keep his penis erect with occasional thrusts while he stimulates the woman's clitoris; when the woman feels she is on the cusp of orgasm, she can ask the man to speed up his thrusting/arousal, so that they can enjoy climaxing together. Just keep in mind that achieving simultaneous orgasms can sometimes take quite a bit of practice, and is not necessarily the be-all and end-all of sexual experiences.

Is It Okay to Have Intercourse During My Period?

A lot of women wonder if it's safe and/or healthy to have intercourse while they are menstruating. Some are open to it, but worry that their partners will be "turned off." Other women report that their partners are eager to do so but that they feel uncomfortable or embarrassed by the idea. Ultimately, the decision whether to have intercourse during menstruation is a personal one: some couples do, some couples don't, and others do sometimes. Those who refrain may do so for any number of reasons: religious or cultural prohibitions, fear of things getting "too messy," or simply because it's not aesthetically pleasing to them. Generally speaking, there is nothing wrong or dangerous about it—so if you and your partner are both into it, there is no reason not to go for it. Some couples may even find sex during menstruation particularly enjoyable as there is no risk whatsoever of pregnancy. Others find they enjoy the extra lubrication that comes with the onset of the menses. (Though it is worth noting that because blood is acidic, it may cause irritation.)

One thing to be aware of is that having intercourse during one's period is likely to intensify the bleeding, at least initially. Although it may seem like an increase in blood volume, it is merely the result of the penis tapping against the cervix and uterus during thrusting and "shaking out" menstrual blood. This is nothing to be alarmed about; it's simply a mechanical issue that's unrelated to your uterine lining or the hormones associated with menstruation. The good news is that you may be done with your period sooner than usual.

———

His erection and you

Of course, you can't have an honest discussion about intercourse without talking about the penis—more specifically, the erect or "hard" penis, which is the result of the penile shaft filling with blood during male sexual arousal. In its erect state, the penis enters the vagina (with or without the woman guiding it into place, which we'll discuss in greater detail below) and commences a rhythmic, thrusting motion, guided by the man's arousal.

When it comes to thrusting, women often ask us, "How deep should the penis go?" The answer is as deep as a woman's vaginal depth allows and as deep as the man's desire guides him—but most importantly, *as deep as is comfortable for you*. Another question we're frequently asked is, "Should the penis fully exit and then re-enter the vagina during thrusting, going all the way in and then all the way out repeatedly?" The answer here is that while each woman will have her individual preferences, the vast majority find the back-and-forth rocking movement much more comfortable—and, for some, quite pleasurable!—when the penis remains inside the vagina for the duration of intercourse.

Naturally, how long intercourse lasts is also an important matter to consider. And the sometimes typical response—"until the man is done"—should *never* be taken as a given. As the "hostess" to the penis, remember that you can always tell your guest when he's overstaying his welcome! It's not unusual for a man to try to engage in thrusting for as long as possible in an effort to slow down his path to climax. While there is nothing wrong with either partner seeking to enhance his or her pleasure, a potential side-effect here is that a woman's vaginal lubrication (whether natural or artificial) may begin to dry out, leading to pain or discomfort. In such cases, it may be worthwhile to take a break and/or take a moment to apply additional lubrication, either to the vaginal opening or directly into the vagina, using an applicator. However, if you find that intercourse is dragging on beyond your level of physical or emotional comfort, there is absolutely nothing wrong with kindly, but firmly, letting your partner know that you're ready to call it a night.

In addition to the question of how long the thrusting motion of intercourse should last, it's also worth considering the style and speed of thrusting that you prefer, which like all sexual preferences, will depend on how you're feeling during any given encounter. This is not a time to be shy! Respectfully let your partner know if you want him to move slower, faster, harder, softer, or any other way that you think might enhance your comfort. If you've recently given birth or undergone surgery, for example, it may take some time before you are able to engage in intercourse again—and when you do, a gentle approach will probably work best, at least initially. After all, the velocity of the penis tapping against the cervix can at times feel intense or overwhelming; there is nothing wrong with letting your partner know if you need to slow things down. It's also worth taking into account the particular character of your partner's penis: if it is curved, bent, unusually long or thick, or especially short, specific modifications may be in order.

What If He Loses His Erection?

While most men in most situations will be able to achieve and sustain an erection, there may be instances when this is not the case. Indeed, if you've been in this situation, as many of us will be at one time or another, you may have asked yourself some version of the following questions:

▶ "Is it my fault that he lost his erection?"

▶ "What am I doing wrong?"

▶ "Is it my responsibility to make sure he stays hard?"

▶ "Is it fair for my boyfriend to blame me?"

▶ "Does it mean he doesn't love me anymore?"

▶ "Is this a sign that he doesn't think I'm sexy?"

Because this is such a prevalent, yet rarely discussed, subject, let us address these questions one by one: No, it is not your fault if your partner loses his erection. No, you have not done anything wrong. No, it is not your responsibility to make sure he stays hard. No, it is not fair for your boyfriend (or anyone else, for that matter) to blame you. No, it does not mean he doesn't love you or that you are not sexy. Whew. Now that we've cleared that up, let's talk about what *is* true.

The fact of the matter is that although "it takes two to tango," as it were, each partner, whether male or female, is responsible for his or her own personal sexual satisfaction. This means that it is not your "job" to ensure your partner's arousal (and subsequent orgasm) any more than it is his "job" to ensure yours. What each of us is responsible for is communicating our wants and needs in a respectful way, and letting our partner know what he or she can do to help us achieve sexual pleasure (which may—or may not—result in orgasm). If anyone tries to tell you otherwise, or if your partner tries to shame, blame, or belittle you, it may be worth considering whether he is in fact an appropriate sexual partner for you.

Sadly, it is still widely perceived that a woman is responsible for a man's sexual pleasure and that it is her job to ensure his satisfaction, an idea that remains deeply rooted in our cultural perceptions of sexuality and gender roles. Indeed, some traditions and religions enforce this imbalance by implying that a man will suffer—physically, spiritually, or both—if he is not adequately sexually "serviced." Meanwhile, medical school curricula still tend to educate future health professionals about sexuality from a male point of view, with only passing references to female sexuality. This is to say nothing of the media, which continuously bombards women with the message that they must look and act sexy at all times in order to attract and keep a man's attention.

While this widespread attitude is unlikely to change overnight, one of our goals in writing this book is to educate women that there is another way to see things. By taking responsibility for our own sexuality, and encouraging our partners to do the same, we can all be part of a change.

———

Guiding the penis

Generally speaking, the erect penis has a built-in GPS and can find its way into the vagina without any guidance, aided by the V-shape of the pelvic bones by the genitals. However, the question of whether or not a woman ought to specifically guide, or even insert, the penis directly into her vagina, is a question that comes up often, particularly among those who are new to intercourse. As in so many other areas of sexual behavior, there is no right or wrong. Rather, it's a classic case of "different strokes for different folks," taking into account your preferences, your partner's preferences, and your levels of experience.

Some women always guide, while others never do, or only do with some partners and/or in certain positions. Meanwhile, some men prefer to guide themselves, while others find they enjoy being "ushered" into place, and that their partner's touch adds to their sexual arousal and sense of intimacy. On a practical level, women with especially sensitive vaginal tissue, whether due to menopause, radiation treatments or conditions such as vaginismus or dyspareunia are likely to prefer taking a more "hands on" approach, which will help to minimize pain and irritation.

Whether or not you choose to guide your partner's penis, you want to be sure that it is sufficiently erect—in other words, very hard—before you attempt intercourse. The reason for this is straightforward: It is simply impossible for a soft or floppy penis to fit into the vagina. Unfortunately, many less-than-experienced couples do not realize this, leading to hours (and sadly, sometimes years) of needless frustration, hurt feelings, and confusion about why things "aren't working." Keep in mind that just because a man may think or feel that his penis is fully erect, and therefore prepared for intercourse, does not necessarily mean it is: sometimes there is a disconnect between his perception and his actual physical state. Thus, when we talk about guiding the penis, it's also worth considering giving the penis some extra stimulation if necessary, whether with your hand or with your mouth, to ensure that your partner is in fact ready. This simple step can go a long way in terms of ensuring that the experience is successful and satisfying for both of you.

What If I Bleed?

Occasionally, a woman may discover that she's had some bleeding following vaginal intercourse, whether in the form of active bleeding or as "spotting" on her underwear or bedsheets. While the sight of unexpected blood can understandably be alarming, in most cases the bleeding and/or spotting is perfectly benign, and may be caused by:

▶ Irritation as a result of vaginal dryness and/or insufficient lubrication.
▶ The stretching or tearing of hymeneal tissue if intercourse is still a new activity for you.
▶ The weakening of vaginal tissue as a result of the estrogen depletion associated with menopause or cancer treatments.
▶ Leftover menstrual blood (if your period has recently ended)

which was shaken out by the tapping motion of the penis against the uterus.

▸ Vaginismus or dyspareunia, which causes your vaginal opening (introitus) to tighten, leading to chafing and possibly tearing, or vulvodynia, characterized by micro tears of that area.

So, before you panic and imagine the worst, consider if any of the above might apply. Also, remember that a drop of blood, when mixed with other fluids such as lubrication or semen, may give the impression of more blood than there actually is. As always, seek medical advice to ensure genital health.

His orgasm

While most men are able to achieve orgasm through intercourse without any problems, for others there may be challenges, the most common of which are premature ejaculation and delayed ejaculation. In the case of premature ejaculation, a man climaxes and releases semen immediately upon arousal and/or penetration. Understandably, this can prompt feelings of failure and disappointment for the man, but it can also be equally frustrating for his partner, who may be left wondering what she did "wrong" or if it's her "fault." Without a doubt, this challenge will put great stress on the relationship. The affected man should consider medical consultation, sexual therapy, medication, as well as psychotherapy as this is a psychophysical condition and needs to be addressed as such. One possible solution for the couple is to follow a premature ejaculation with another round of intercourse. This will entail waiting until the man is able to achieve an erection again, known as the "refractory period," which typically lasts anywhere from five minutes to an hour, depending on the individual.

While premature ejaculation effectively puts an end to intercourse before it's begun, delayed ejaculation can drag out the sexual act for "what seems like forever," as one of our patients put it. Because a man who experiences delayed ejaculation (also known as retarded ejaculation) has great difficulty climaxing, his "solution" is often to simply continue thrusting, blind to the passing of time and his partner's comfort, resulting in an experience that's exhausting (and joyless) for them both. Not to mention the toll it takes on a woman's body. As the above patient told us, "After forty minutes of his trying to achieve his 'goal,' I feel all ripped up." While going along despite her own discomfort initially seemed like the easiest path to take, the "doing it for him" approach, as we like to call it, generally tends to result in resentment, and ultimately, a reluctance to engage sexually. Instead, we recommend the following solutions, which are far more sustainable:

- Have your partner pull out temporarily during intercourse so you can apply additional lubrication to your vaginal opening or into the vagina using a vaginal applicator, or both.
- Engage in outercourse (oral sex or dry sex) for his arousal, then use intercourse for the final few moments/climax.
- Take a break from intercourse to stimulate your partner manually.
- Take a break from intercourse and ask your partner to stimulate himself. (Remember: the responsibility for his sexual satisfaction is not solely yours!)
- It's also okay to let your partner know if you want to call it quits for now. If he so wishes, he can continue with his own self-stimulation.

Finally, if your partner is struggling with either premature or delayed ejaculation, he should seek medical attention from his family physician or urologist. If all illnesses or infections have been ruled out, he may want to consider enlisting the help of a licensed psychotherapist or sex therapist to help him address the underlying problem.

Do Women Ejaculate?

Female ejaculation is another one of those misconceptions floating around. In males, ejaculation is the expulsion of sperm and seminal fluid, the white fluid collectively known as "ejaculate." Biologically speaking, it is the pressure of the ejaculation plus the swimming ability of the sperm that ultimately facilitate its journey into the cervix en route to meeting a just-ovulated egg in the fallopian tubes for fertilization and conception (hence, pregnancy). While some women claim to have experienced female ejaculation, recent studies, including anatomical imaging, have shown that there is no ejaculatory mechanism in the female genitals. So what are these women experiencing? There are several possibilities:

▸ She is a heavy lubricator and may experience some "leakage"
▸ The urethra (urine tube) expels residual urine
▸ The muscle contraction associated with orgasm releases residual mucus/lubrication from the vagina and/or the uterus
▸ The expulsion of fluids from the paraurethral ducts/Skene glands, which are mucus glands in the wall of the lower urethra that are often referred to as the 'female prostate'
▸ Any combination of the above

Masturbation: Sex Just for You

While masturbation is a perfectly natural, normal, and necessary part of being a fully developed sexual being, many women remain reluctant to engage in it, let alone talk about it. Others are prohibited from practicing it for religious reasons. Some women associate masturbation exclusively with men, erroneously assuming that it's an activity reserved for sex-obsessed teenagers or sex-starved older men. The truth, however, is that self-stimulation, as we prefer to call it, is a wonderful way to learn about your own sexuality without worrying about anyone else's preferences, judgments, or preconceived notions. It is, in other words, a time to create a safe and private space that is just for you, in which all you have to focus on is what—depending on your mood—relaxes you, turns you on, and/or brings you to climax.

Contrary to popular belief, female masturbation does not necessarily involve the vagina at all. While vaginal stimulation, whether with a vibrator, dildo, or finger may enhance the experience, self-stimulation is primarily about the clitoris, which is the woman's main sexual organ. Regardless of your age, sexual orientation, or relationship status, self-stimulation is without a doubt the single best way to learn about what feels good to you and what kind of touch—hard, soft, fast, slow, up-and-down, circular, or just about anything else—excites you most. For women who have never before experienced orgasm, or for those who believe they are simply unable to do so, taking the time to educate yourself about your sexuality in this way is invaluable, particularly if previous attempts to achieve orgasm with a partner have ended in disappointment and frustration.

If you are just getting started, we recommend finding a quiet time and place, such as the shower, bath, or your own bed, and shutting off any external distractions, including electronic devices. You may want to turn off the lights to create a calm environment, or do it before falling asleep, and perhaps even do some deep breathing to help you relax. You may or may not want to experiment with the use of a lubricant or vibrator; whether or not you choose to do so, remember to make sure your clitoris remains sufficiently lubricated, which not only helps with arousal but will also prevent any uncomfortable irritation or chafing. Some women like to fantasize, while others don't. Of those who do, some use porn specifically designed for women, while others prefer to just let their mind wander. There is no right or wrong—the key is to find whatever works for you.

If you are currently in a relationship, you may or may not choose to share with your partner what you've learned. If you feel comfortable, you may consider showing him or her how you like to be touched, whether using your own hand or guiding theirs. It's worth mentioning that a mature and supportive partner has no need to feel "jealous" of your ability to satisfy yourself sexually, and should only encourage you in your ongoing journey of self-discovery.

Manual Sex

As in the case of self-stimulation, when we talk about manual sex for women, we are not necessarily talking about vaginal stimulation (also known as "fingering"), but rather, clitoral stimulation. Because it is the clitoris, and not the vagina, that is the primary female sexual organ, this is where the action is, so to speak. Whether as a stand-alone activity, or as a lead-in to oral or vaginal intercourse, manual sex—by which we mean your partner stroking, rubbing, or massaging your clitoris with their hand—is a safe, low-risk way for your partner to give to you sexually. (Of course, manual sex is often a two-way street, with partners taking turns. So after you have climaxed, you may want to return the favor.) Because there is no need for birth control nor the up-close intimacy of oral sex, many women find that they are able to enjoy manual stimulation freely. It's also worth noting that it's an activity that women who suffer from vaginismus are also able to enjoy, since it requires no vaginal penetration.

As with other items on the sexual menu, let your own pleasure be your guide and keep your partner in the loop! If you want him or her to touch you in a specific way, say so, or simply guide their hand. Hopefully, you will already have an idea of what you like based on your own experiences with self-stimulation. If your partner goes straight for your vagina, with the assumption that a marathon session of "fingering" will lead you to orgasm, gently redirect him or ask if he would like to be shown what you like. Trust us: a partner who is interested in your pleasure will be only too happy to oblige!

When You're Not In The Mood

When we talk about the sexual menu, it's also worth talking about those times when nothing on the menu seems to interest you. Just like there may be times when you visit a beloved restaurant and even your favorite dishes just don't sound appealing, so too there will be days (or nights), sometimes for stretches at a time, when you're just not in the mood for sexual contact. Provided this is not part of a longstanding, deeply ingrained pattern of avoiding sex with your partner, it is perfectly natural to cycle in and out of sexual interest. While this is true of both genders, it is particularly true for women, who need to know that it does not mean anything is wrong with their relationship. So what do you do if your partner's feeling it and you're not?

In such situations, something we call "bartering" can come in handy. By bartering we mean suggesting an alternative to sexual activity, but one that will still facilitate intimacy and closeness. For example, you might tell your partner that at the moment you'd prefer a back rub or a foot massage or that the two of you go for a nighttime stroll around the block. In other cases, you can explain that you are willing to sexually satisfy him, say with oral or manual sex, even if you're not in the mood for anything sexual in return, and ask for an "IOU" to be redeemed at another time of your choosing.

Dry Sex

"Dry sex" or "humping" is a form of non-penetrative sexual activity that takes place with both partners fully or partially clothed. It may involve lying on top of each other and moving in an arousing, rhythmic motion, or it may entail the rubbing or touching of genitals over the underwear. If arousal is sustained for long enough, it can even result in orgasm, even though there is no direct contact. If done solo, it may be against a pillow or a folded towel, etc.

Though typically associated with teenagers or couples with limited sexual experience, dry sex can be a safe—and, for some, very exciting—sexual outlet. For some, it is the only acceptable option due to religious or cultural restrictions against premarital sex, while for others it can be a healthy, risk-free option if direct genital contact is ill-advised due to a herpes outbreak or other active sexually transmitted infection.

Oral Sex: Do or Don't?

"Is everyone having oral sex except for me?" Not quite. And yet, given the frequency with which it's discussed in popular culture, it's easy to understand why it may sometimes seem that way. The fact of the matter is that oral sex—whether given or received—is ultimately a personal choice, one that every individual must make for herself. While some of us may have been taught that oral sex is "wrong" or somehow "unclean," the truth is that it is a perfectly normal and healthy way of sharing sexual pleasure with another person. It can also offer the opportunity to learn more about what exactly turns *you* on as well as how to satisfy your partner's most intimate desires. Some

women find they are particularly turned on by being the sole focus of a partner's attention, as in the act of cunnilingus; conversely, others discover they enjoy focusing completely on their partners' gratification, which can offer its own sense of empowerment and fulfillment.

As an added bonus, oral sex carries no risk of pregnancy, which in and of itself may help couples who do not wish to conceive to feel more relaxed. However, it is still crucial to remember that when it comes to receiving and/or giving oral sex, *safe sex practices still apply*.

It is also worth mentioning here that there is nothing wrong with choosing to refrain from oral sex, whether for personal, cultural, or religious reasons, any more than there is something wrong with choosing to enjoy it. We encourage women to make such decisions based on their own beliefs and preferences rather than from a place of fear. While it is, of course, always your choice to say "no," it may be worthwhile to first give it a try, particularly in the context of a safe and supportive relationship, where there is room for trial and error. It's also okay to be in the mood sometimes and not others. If you feel like you are open to experimenting with oral sex but are not quite ready to do so, share your thoughts and concerns with your partner. You may determine that even if it is not something you are ready to embark on today, an open dialogue may help set the stage for trying it out in the future.

How to Have Oral Sex Safely

While many of us are well aware that a condom is required for vaginal intercourse that takes place outside of an established, STI-tested monogamous relationship, what's less widely known is that sexually transmitted infections can be transmitted just as easily during oral-genital contact. So, if you plan to perform oral sex on your male partner, make sure he first puts on a condom—just make sure the condom does not contain spermicide, which although non-toxic, will not taste too good and may even have a slightly numbing effect on your mouth due to the chemicals they contain to prolong a man's arousal. Flavored condoms, however, are perfectly fine and many women find that performing oral sex is more enjoyable when the penis tastes like a tropical-flavored candy!

When it comes to your partner performing oral sex on you, we recommend first placing what's known as a dental dam on top of the vulva and clitoris. If you're wondering what a dental dam is, it is simply a small square-sized sheet of latex. Originally developed to isolate the affected area during dental procedures, it is now commonly used as a precautionary measure against STIs as well. Of course, it's natural to wonder if cunnilingus will be as enjoyable with a dental dam in place as it is without. The answer is that while the sensations are obviously somewhat different with a piece of latex between you and your partner's tongue, most women report that they are still 100% able to enjoy it. In any event, oral sex with a dental dam is still a far preferable option to dealing with the pain and potential long-term health consequences of contracting an STI.

Finally, it should go without saying that if you or your partner has a cold sore (which is actually an oral strain of herpes) or any other type of oral/dental infection or virus, oral sex should be avoided until you or your partner has received proper medical treatment. It is always within your rights to let an affected partner know that you will postpone sexual activity until his infection is under control. Similarly, if you are the one affected, it's okay to tell your partner, "I'm not going to engage until I'm healthy."

Oral sex: for her

When performed on a woman, oral sex entails her partner moving his or her mouth and tongue on or around her clitoris, which may or may not culminate in orgasm. Officially known as cunnilingus (in Latin, cunnus means "vulva" and lingus means "to lick"), it is also referred to as "going down," "eating out," or any other number of (sometimes derogatory) slang. While some couples enthusiastically embrace this activity, others are more hesitant, and some may dismiss it altogether, some for religious reasons, others citing concerns about it being "dirty" or "gross." We, however, could not disagree more—and as with a range of other sexual activities, we encourage couples not to knock it till they try it!

Why? Because there is much to recommend about it. For one, the built-in lubrication provided by saliva is not only extremely pleasurable for many women, it can also help reduce the risk of dryness or irritation that may accompany intercourse. For another, the tongue is typically able to move at different speeds (fast, slow, or any combination) and in various motions (up and down, side to side, in circles), based on what his or her partner finds arousing at any given moment. In fact, some women find that the sustained pressure of tongue-to-genital contact helps them to achieve orgasm in a way that few sexual activities can match.

Nevertheless, we still meet many women who report feeling shy, nervous, or embarrassed about being on the receiving end of the oral sex equation. Indeed, when it comes to oral sex, it's not uncommon for our patients to tell us, *"I'm more likely to give than to receive," "I'm fine with his penis touching my vagina, but not his mouth,"* or *"I feel okay doing it to him, but I don't want him to do it to me."* Unfortunately, the reasons our patients give typically fall under the category of not feeling "clean down there"—including embarrassment about how their genitals will look, taste, and smell, as well as concern about the presence of natural discharge. For others of us, who have been conditioned throughout our lives to be "givers" and not "takers," the very notion of lying back and allowing another to devote his energies exclusively to our pleasure can pose its own set of emotional challenges. Perhaps we feel we're being "selfish" or that we don't deserve that kind of attention.

When it comes to receiving oral sex, we like to remind women that for some of us, the process of embracing our vulvas without unfounded worries is a learning curve—one that takes time, gentleness, and patience. If you find the idea of letting your partner get "too close" to your genitals, or if you find yourself struggling with feelings of shame about your body in general, it may be helpful to discuss these concerns directly with your partner, or with a trusted friend or counselor. The following are some additional tips that may help to make being the "receiver" more enjoyable:

- As long as you shower regularly and practice basic genital hygiene, there is no reason to feel ashamed about how you smell. The vagina, like the penis, has its own scent. The goal is to be clean, not sterile. Of course, if you have a urinary tract infection, an STI, or vaginal infection, it makes sense to refrain from sexual activity until it has been properly treated; discuss with your physician whether your partner needs to be treated as well.

- If you are still concerned about your scent, or if you are simply interested in adding variety to your sexual repertoire, try using a flavored lubricant, which will also provide clitoral lubrication.
- Guide your partner! Don't be afraid to tell him or her what you like, either verbally or with your hand. Let your partner know if you prefer him or her to move his or her tongue slower, faster, softer, harder, etc.
- Remember your partner's comfort. Even when you are on the receiving end, oral sex is still a two-way street. While it's vital to communicate your preferences, your partner's comfort is also important. Help to ensure that his or her neck and mouth joints are in a satisfactory position.
- Let go of the pressure to "succeed." Cunnilingus need not culminate in orgasm each and every time. Together, you and your partner may determine how long—or how short—a session will last and whether it will take place in conjunction with other sexual activities. Particularly if you're new to oral sex, it's worth remembering that there's no pressure to go from zero to a hundred miles an hour in one session!

Oral sex: for him

Compared to women, men are typically less hesitant about receiving oral sex, and most males will make no secret of the pleasure they take in it. Commonly referred to as a "blowjob," the act of fellatio involves the licking and sucking, often in a rhythmic, up-and-down motion, of the penile shaft and/or scrotum. This may or may not include manual stimulation (i.e., the use of one's hand); it may be performed as "the main act" or serve as a prelude to intercourse, with some men preferring to enjoy it on its own terms, while others use it to build momentum and strengthen their erection for other activities.

As with most other "dishes" on the sexual menu, fellatio can last anywhere from a few moments to as long as a partner is willing to partake. However, be aware that if a man is in the mood to prolong his pleasure, it can lead to jaw pain for his partner. This is not at all uncommon, so if you find yourself in this situation, speak up! It's okay to let your partner know if the activity has progressed beyond your level of comfort. Participating in a particular sexual activity should never mean putting yourself in a situation that causes you pain, physical or otherwise. You can suggest taking a break, moving on to another form of stimulation for him or giving him a chance to stimulate you for a while. Remember: being the "giver" should never equal suffering in silence. Below are some of the other concerns women typically share with us when it comes to performing oral sex . . .

- **"I don't want him to ejaculate in my mouth."** If you don't enjoy swallowing your partner's ejaculate when he reaches orgasm, you are not alone. Despite what your partner may tell you (or what he's seen in media), ingesting his semen is not a given, but a choice that is yours—and yours only—to make. If you choose not to swallow, as many women do, you and your partner can develop a signal so that you can move your mouth away when he anticipates his climax, or, if you so choose, you can let the semen collect in your mouth and then spit it into a tissue or towel. Alternatively, you might consider using flavored condoms, which are made for this very reason. With practice, most couples are able to come up with a system that takes both parties' comfort into consideration.
- **"My boyfriend says I have to give him oral sex."** The answer to this is simple: There is no such thing as "have to." While there's nothing wrong with your boyfriend or partner or husband wanting oral sex, deciding whether to engage in any sexual activity is always a decision that involves both of you.
- **"What if my partner is uncircumcised?"** Whether or not your partner is circumcised, it is very important that the penis is clean before commencing with oral sex. So if it's on the agenda, give him a (gentle) nudge to take a shower if he hasn't already! Men who are uncircumcised will need to take special care to make sure that their foreskin has been properly cleaned and that there is no residue hiding underneath.
- **"My boyfriend wants to perform oral sex on my anus, but I don't think it's safe."** There is nothing wrong with oral-to-anal sex, which is also known as analingus or rimming, as long as (1) You feel

comfortable trying it (2) He stops if and when you say so, and (3) You practice basic hygiene. This means thoroughly cleaning the anal area beforehand to remove residual fecal matter, and ensuring that your partner does not have cold sores, Hepatitis, E-Coli, Intestinal parasites, Sexually Transmitted infections (STIs), or other transmittable viruses that can be spread through oral-to-anal sex. If he performs oral sex on your genitals during the same session, it is fine to move from the genitals to the anus, but NEVER the reverse, which could also introduce harmful bacteria into your vulva and/or vaginal canal. To reduce the risk of infection, it is recommended to use a barrier between mouth and anus, i.e. Sheer® GLYDE dam, plastic wrap, dental dam, or a cut-up condom.

Anal Intercourse

Anal sex, which involves the insertion of the penis into the rectum, was once a rarely talked-about phenomenon, in part because of its association with male homosexual sex, but also because any reference to the anus tends to conjure up images of defection and elimination, and therefore, shame. In recent years, as male homosexuality has increasingly become more accepted, and a wider variety of sexual options have entered the mainstream cultural conversation, so too has discussion of heterosexual anal sex, along with the awareness that it is much more common among male-female couples than once was believed. While some women undoubtedly enjoy it, and others remain curious, our experience shows that most feel hesitant to engage in the practice, with some feeling outright disgusted by the prospect. The reasons they cite range anywhere from religious prohibitions to the perception of it being "dirty," "degrading," or simply "unnatural."

We, however, maintain that as long as it involves two consenting adults, and as long as hygienic and safer sex precautions are taken, there is no reason why anal intercourse can't have its place on the sexual menu. For those who are interested, whether it becomes a regular part of your sexual repertoire or you are merely looking to try it out, it's vital to keep the following guidelines in mind:

- Lubricate, lubricate, lubricate. Because the anal canal was not expressly designed for sexual activity and does not self-lubricate in the way that the vagina does, anal intercourse mandates generous use of lubrication. Not only will this help to ensure that the experience is as comfortable and pleasurable as possible, it will also help to facilitate penetration, thereby reducing the chance of any painful tearing or soreness. As always, we recommend a non-irritating water-based formula rather than an oil-based version, which can wreak havoc with a latex condom. Which brings us to our next point . . .

- Take safer sex precautions. Just because you can't get pregnant through anal intercourse doesn't mean you don't need to use a condom! Unless you are in a monogamous STI-tested relationship of long-standing, it is vital that a condom be worn during anal intercourse, as STIs and other infections can be easily transmitted via the rectum.

- Practice sensible hygiene. While it is okay to transition from vaginal intercourse to anal intercourse, the reverse is never advisable. The reason? Anal bacteria is not compatible with the vaginal environment, and if introduced, will almost certainly lead to infections, discomfort, and other complications.

- Vary anal intercourse with other sexual activities. While we are all for anal intercourse—provided that you enjoy it and take the above recommendations into account—medically speaking, there are consequences to be aware of if you engage in it frequently. Repetitive anal intercourse may result in the stretching of the anal sphincter, which can lead to fecal incontinence. Thus, we recommend reserving the activity as a once-in-a-while addition to your sexual repertoire, and to make sure you're enjoying other forms of sexual contact as well, which do not carry the same risks of long-term impact on your body. If anal stimulation is something that both you and your partner take pleasure in, an alternative to penis-anal intercourse is for your partner to stimulate your anal area with his or her finger, tongue ("rimming"), or a dildo—as long as you remember to practice proper hygiene.

One final note on the subject: Sadly, we have at times met with women who have been forced by their partners to engage in anal sex against their will. In other cases, we have seen patients who were simply unable to say NO to their partners' insistent requests, and in some instances, outright demands. Furthermore, as a result of the prevalent misconception that anal sex is not "real sex," and therefore doesn't "count" when it comes to issues like preserving virginity and premarital intercourse, some men (and women) see it as the only option for sexual contact outside of marriage, regardless of whether or not the woman is comfortable with the idea. Needless to say, our aim is to remind all women that whether or not to have anal intercourse—and, for that matter, any form of sexual contact—is always up to them. Our hope and prayer is that all women will one day have the freedom to exercise their rights to make their own sexual choices.

Lesbian and Bisexual Sexuality

While some women maintain an exclusive attraction to men throughout the course of their lifetime and others maintain an exclusive attraction to women, others may go through periods of questioning and experimentation, engaging in relationships with both men and women at different points in their lives. Despite what some of us may have been taught to believe, exploration and experimentation are a natural and necessary part of our development as human beings. Whether we ultimately choose to identify as straight, gay, bisexual, transgender—or whether we prefer not to place a label on our sexuality at all—we believe that every woman's path to discovering her sexual identity is legitimate. If you are struggling with some of these questions, we encourage you to give yourself the permission to sort through it, whether with the help of a psychotherapist, sexual counselor, or a trusted friend.

Although sexual relationships between women may, in some ways, be easier to negotiate as a result of the couple sharing the same sexual template, many of the principles discussed above still apply: the importance of making your own needs and desires known, maintaining a general openness to trying new things, and learning to communicate respectfully and effectively with your partner. Wherever you find yourself on the sexual spectrum, the most important thing is that you are able to express yourself freely.

In terms of the sexual menu, lesbian and bisexual couples have many of the same options as a heterosexual couple, with the obvious exception of a biological penis. However, if two women are interested in exploring the pleasures of penetration, whether in the form of vaginal or anal sex, there are a range of sexual accessories, including standard dildos and strap-on dildos, which many women use to add variety to their sex lives. Though some lesbian couples are adverse to such accessories out of a conviction that they imply the "superiority" of heterosexual sex and are used to mimic it, we encourage same-sex couples to take a non-judgmental approach, and to enjoy whatever it is that they find exciting.

When it comes to same-sex sexual relationships, our one word of caution is to remember that women can transmit and/or receive Sexually Transmitted infections to and from other women, so taking safer sex precautions still applies. This is also true for bisexual women, who may have contracted an STI from a male partner, even without realizing it. While it may be easy to forget in the heat of the moment, unless you are in an exclusive STI-tested relationship, it is never just the two of you in the bedroom. So if you are engaging in oral sex outside of a monogamous relationship, we recommend using a dental dam until both you and your partner have been tested.

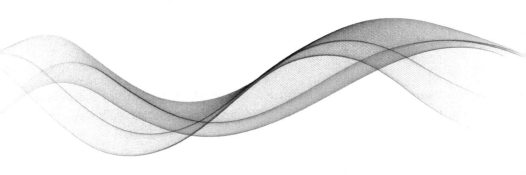

Chapter Five

Beyond the "Oohs" and "Aahs"

Owning Your Orgasm

Arousing the Clitoris

Any discussion of female orgasm must begin with an introduction to the clitoris (see Chapter One) and how it works. It is important to remember that unlike the vagina, the clitoris is not self-lubricating and thus is prone to chafing irritations upon prolonged and/or rough contact. While the saliva present during oral sex usually provides sufficient lubrication, in the case of manual sex, dry sex, and the use of toys, we encourage women (and/or their partners) to apply lubricant to the clitoris, especially if you are prone to discomfort.

While vaginal stimulation may be pleasurable for some women, it is clitoral stimulation that is necessary for sexual arousal and orgasm. Direct clitoral stimulation may be achieved through one or a combination of the following methods:

- **Masturbation:** stimulation on your own or with your partner's hand. May or may not include "fingering"
- **Dry sex**

- Oral sex
- **Vibrator:** used on the clitoris, or inside the vagina, or both

Indirect clitoral stimulation may occur when the base of the penis during intercourse rubs the clitoris and inner lips in just the right way.

How do I Know if I'm Having an Orgasm?

An orgasm is a series of muscle contractions of the pelvic diaphragm that signal the climax of sexual excitation. Orgasm is typically experienced as a building up of pleasurable sensation in and around the clitoris and inside the vagina, culminating in a physiological sense of release. While some women are able to clearly identify—and enjoy—their orgasms, others have difficulty determining whether the pleasure they're experiencing is "it."

In some women, orgasm may be accompanied by shortness of breath or a shaking sensation. Other women may experience a wave of warmth or flush, a twitching of the muscles inside the vagina, faint or strong, accompanied by a sense of euphoria. Some women may moan or groan, some may scream in ecstasy, while others may remain absolutely still. This variety is natural, and there is no right or wrong.

Your orgasm doesn't know if you are single or married, young or old, fulfilled or frustrated. It is simply a physiological ability to reach a state of excitement—with or without a partner, with or without sexual toys, with or without romance. An orgasm can be a strictly physical experience, or it can be an emotional one as well. It can be a way of taking time to connect with yourself, to indulge in fantasy, or a special moment to share with another person.

We often see women in our clinic who are confused about where in the female anatomy the orgasm originates. This confusion can sometimes lead to the all-too-common case in which a woman is experiencing orgasms without even realizing it. Susie, a single, 22-year-old college student, had come to us for sex counseling. As part of an intake of her sexual history, we asked Susie if she was able to bring herself to orgasm by masturbating. Susie looked at us, obviously confused. Eventually she mumbled, "I really don't like to put my finger in my vagina." When we explained that the clitoris is outside the vagina and that fingering is not mandatory for arousal, she said, "Oh, yeah, I bring myself to orgasm all the time."

What If I Can't Have an Orgasm?

The inability to achieve orgasm is rarely rooted in physical causes. Contrary to common opinion, the ability to orgasm is also rarely affected by medication, including anti-depressant or anti-anxiety medication, unless taken in very high doses. If you find that you cannot have an orgasm, either by yourself or with a partner, you may want to seek professional consultation. Speak with your primary care physician or gynecologist or ask for a referral to a sex therapist.

The Myth of Vaginal Orgasm

One of the most common questions we get is "Am I the only one who cannot climax (orgasm) when his penis is inside me (intercourse)?"

The answer is no, not at all—but let us explain. As mentioned above, the clitoris, and not the vagina, is the primary female erogenous structure, the anatomical parallel to the male's penis. The vagina, on the other hand, is not an erogenous zone per se, but a passageway. (Think about it this way: if your vagina were your primary erogenous zone, then every gynecological exam or tampon insertion would be an erotic experience!) It is clitoral stimulation—direct or indirect—that is necessary for female sexual arousal. So unless you are among the rare subset of women whose pelvic alignment is such that your partner's penis rubs your clitoris in an arousing way during intercourse, direct clitoral stimulation will be necessary if you wish to orgasm simultaneously with your partner. You can use your hand, your partner's hand, or alternatively, a vibrator. Clitoral stimulation can be started before the penis is inside you (foreplay) or when it is already inside you, in which case your partner will have to hold back on climaxing in order to coordinate your orgasmic rhythms.

The myth that most women can reach orgasm through intercourse alone leads to unneeded feelings of disappointment and inadequacy. Sadly, the misconception that unless you have a vaginal orgasm you're not having a "real" orgasm or the "ultimate" orgasm, leads some women to doubt themselves and their sexuality. Some women may even come to medicalize their so-called problem, convinced that there is something "wrong" with them—a position that, unfortunately, some healthcare providers may validate. The truth is, most women simply do not experience vaginal orgasm. We have seen many patients attempt to fulfill this ideal, with frustrating results that are harmful to their self-esteem and in turn, negatively impact their sex lives. This perceived sense of failure also impacts the woman's partner, often leading to a vicious cycle of frustration and blame. The fact is most women cannot climax through intercourse, so if this is your experience, you can consider yourself in normal, healthy company.

The Quest for a 'Good' Orgasm

Women often come to us with the complaint, "I do not have good orgasms!," which begs the question: *what is a "good" orgasm?* A lack of adequate sexual education combined with a bombardment of media images leave many people—women and men alike—confused about what kind of orgasms they or their partners "should" be having. The following letter, which we received from the husband of a former patient, illustrates how this confusion, together with a lack of communication, can end up causing needless frustration:

> *I still have not been able to give my wife sensual pleasure during sexual intimacy. I tried many suggestions mentioned in the books as well as what you taught us, but her body just does not feel the sensation of pleasure that I expect. Is there anything I can do about it?*

Knowing how subjective individual experiences are in the realm of sexual intimacy, we arranged for a discussion with the couple to clarify the situation. In our meeting, the wife reported that she was having orgasms just fine. While they weren't the kind of "big" orgasms typically portrayed in the media, she felt both emotionally and sexually satisfied and reported to her husband that she was, in fact, very happy with their sex life. It soon emerged that her husband had been expecting his wife to feel the same kind of explosive orgasms that he'd been experiencing.

As we talked, we explained the differences between male and female orgasms, including the ejaculation factor that is typical to men only. We then explained that both "small" and "big" orgasms—what we coined "minigasms" and "maxigasms" —are normal. Men's orgasms can also vary in intensity from one experience to another. The main thing is each partner's own perception of satisfaction, combined with open, ongoing communication in which these feelings are honestly shared. At the end of the session, both husband and wife left our office relieved, armed with a better understanding of both their sexual expectations and the necessity for more mutual sharing of their experiences.

In other instances, women themselves have come to our office with the complaint that their orgasms are not "good enough." When asked to explain, one woman told us: *"I can orgasm from manual stimulation to the clitoris but they are little orgasms. I can also orgasm from oral sex but they are not big like the ones from a vibrator. I want to have the same powerful orgasm from all activities."*

First, we reminded her that it is perfectly normal to have both mini- and/or maxigasms. We also reminded her that the speed of a vibrator cannot be matched by a hand, a tongue, or the thrust of a penis. There is nothing wrong with enjoying the use of a vibrator, we explained, as long as it does not lead you to diminish or become critical of other forms of sexual arousal.

So, what is a "good" orgasm? By now, we hope you realize there is no such thing. Every woman's orgasm—whether big or small, loud or quiet, with a partner or alone—is unique to her, a gift she can give to herself or share with another if she chooses. We encourage women to explore and discover their own preferred pathway to orgasm, as long as:

- You are not forced into it.
- Lubricant is used as necessary to avoid chaffing.
- You are able to communicate clearly and honestly if you are with a partner ("go faster;" "not too hard;" "I like this").
- Your partner is considerate of your choices/preferences.
- There are no judgments or expectations.
- You are not suffering in silence in order to protect your partner's feelings.

Why Can I Have an Orgasm by Myself but Not with Someone Else?

The first thing you need to know is that if you can have an orgasm by yourself, it means there is nothing wrong with you physically or medically. Instead, the problem is more likely emotional in nature. Perhaps you don't like how your partner stimulates you but you don't know how to tell him. Perhaps you feel forced to "perform" for religious or cultural reasons, and your body shuts down as a result. Maybe you are grappling with unexpressed feelings of anger or resentment toward your partner. We encourage you to explore some of these questions on your own and talk to your partner. You may also want to consult with your healthcare provider or a sex therapist who can help you get to the root of the problem.

Is it Okay to Fake it?

We have often heard women report that as much as their partner tries to bring them to orgasm, they still cannot reach it. Maybe they're just not in the mood at that moment and are unable to say so. Maybe the way their partner is stimulating them simply isn't working, or maybe the woman is worried about oral or manual sex "taking too long." Sometimes, women tell us, it's easier to just fake it and get it over with.

Unfortunately, it is rather common for women to report having faked orgasms. By faking it, we mean conveying to your partner the impression that you've had an orgasm when you haven't; this can range from "oohing and aahing," to a broader repertoire of sounds or motions associated with climax, to verbally affirming to your partner that you "came."

To put it bluntly, faking orgasm is not a good thing. Sexual relationships provide us with an opportunity not only to get to know another person on an intimate level, but also the chance to get to know ourselves sexually. Misrepresenting our experience to our partner deprives us of both opportunities. Of course, the reasons why a woman might choose to fake it vary as described in the following list. What they have in common is that they are all based in some way on feelings of fear, confusion, self-negation, or low self-esteem.

- "I don't know what it's supposed to feel like."
- "I don't know how to communicate to partner what I want."
- "I'm thinking of someone else and want to get it over with."
- "I don't want to disappoint him."
- "I want to make him feel like a man."
- "I want to measure up to his ex."
- "I fake wonderful sex so he won't leave me."

We have also found that anger can play a role in faking orgasms. We often tell women, *If you're angry, spell it out to your partner.* Don't wait for him or her to guess or expect him or her to know what you're upset about, as unexpressed anger will always find its way into the bedroom. Faking also has a way of creating a vicious cycle of distrust and resentment in a relationship. If a woman continuously fakes it, her partner develops a certain understanding of what he or she thinks is pleasurable for her. If she eventually decides to "come clean" and share with her partner what's really going on for her, there is already a history of deceit in place, with the partner left wondering, "Who did I make love to?"

Sexuality is a language, a vital form of self-expression within a romantic partnership. *A lack of honest communication in the sexual realm will always affect the relationship as a whole.* When you are not fully honest, it impacts not only your partner, but your own feelings about the relationship. Instead of coping with your feelings through deceit or avoidance, we encourage you to *help your partner get to know you.* That means sharing with him or her in an open and honest way. Tell your partner how you like to be stimulated and/or guide your partner's hand as he or she stimulates you.

Don't hesitate to speak up—even if you're worried that by *not* faking it, you'll only further disappoint your partner. While it's true that some men feel that if they can't bring a woman to orgasm they are not a "good lover," it is not your job to deny your own experience to protect your partner's feelings. Remember: a sexual relationship is not just about fulfilling your partner's needs, but fulfilling your own. It's about building an authentic and honest relationship with your own body and mind. That means taking time to explore your sexuality (learning what you like) and cultivate your self-esteem (the ability to voice your own preferences).

If you don't know your own preferences, now is the time to find out! After all, if you don't know what you like, how can you expect your partner to? For this reason, we encourage women to learn how to sexually stimulate themselves. For a woman not currently in a relationship, this can be an important tool for reminding herself that she is still a sexual being. For a woman in a relationship, being knowledgeable about her own sexuality makes her more likely to express her desires and needs to her partner. Learning your own preferences—what does or doesn't "turn you on"—is an ongoing, life-long process. You may discover that something that excited you when you were younger no longer does, or, conversely, you may find that as you get older, you're more open to new experiences. For example, we have found that it's not unusual for a woman in her early twenties to be squeamish about receiving oral sex, only to discover some years later how much she enjoys it.

While men tend to be quite clear about their sexual likes and desires, women are sometimes hesitant to speak their minds, opting instead to suffer in silence and/or develop disinterest. Why do so many women continue to act as though they are not equal partners? There are obviously many answers to this question. Ultimately, though, everyone is responsible for his or her own sexual arousal—if you do not tell your partner what you like, how will he or she know?

How Long Should it Take Me to Reach Orgasm?

We get this question a lot. Is an hour the right amount of time or is it too long? Forty-five minutes? Ten? Two? There is no one right answer to this question, no rules or regulations that determine how long it "should" take. Every woman will develop her own rhythm of arousal, which of course may vary depending on her mood, satisfaction with her relationship, and endless other factors.

The Vibrator Question

Since we already brought it up, let's talk about vibrators. Some women feel perfectly comfortable using vibrators, while others shy away from them, perhaps thinking "it's not me," or "why should I need a powered toy to achieve sexual pleasure?" Some cultures and religions object to the use of sexual toys outright. We have also found that some younger, less experienced women may feel that they "don't need them." In other cases, the objection may come from the woman's husband or partner. This may be for religious/cultural reasons, or because he feels inhibited, ashamed, or intimidated. Some men may even see the vibrator as competition, while others simply aren't interested in stretching their sexual comfort zone.

While we respect a woman's right to honor her religious/cultural background, we believe that the vibrator can be a helpful tool in getting to know and exploring your own sexuality, regardless of whether you're single or with a partner. As long as you remember that the clitoris needs lubrication and that vaginal insertion is not required, we encourage women to buy themselves vibrators and enjoy them. (See "tips on choosing a vibrator" in the Resources section at the back of the book.)

While we have seen rare cases in which women use the vibrator to the exclusion of their partners or as a way to distance themselves from relationships (and/or prevent them from moving forward), in most cases vibrators can provide a safe and healthy sexual outlet. Here's what some of our patients have had to say:

"Since my treatment at your center, I have not been with a partner but I have been using a vibrator regularly and it is one of the best investments I have ever made! I am a lot less desperate for intimate company when I can provide such a great pleasure for myself."

"What I found most important was to alternate activity with my husband and with the vibrator so I didn't become so used to the increased stimulation of the vibrator—which, as you say, [other forms of stimulation] cannot match."

"Though I'm only twenty-one, I'd been having issues with sexual arousal. But since you introduced me to the clitoral vibrator, I have learned how to have orgasms on my own. It was so helpful to me, I made a bulk purchase for all the girls in my sorority as a holiday gift!"

Can I Become Addicted to My Vibrator?

While we hear this question not infrequently, we believe that it touches on a much broader issue, which is: Can I become so accustomed to one method of arousal that I am unable to enjoy others? When women share with us their fears of developing such an "addiction," we remind them that the vibrator has no inherent power. It is simply a stimulus that may bring about a preference. Just because a woman may have become accustomed to or developed a preference for the use of a vibrator, does not mean she is not capable of responding to the other forms of stimulation *if she allows herself to*. This is one of those cases where we like to remind women that sexual arousal originates between the ears, not between the legs. In short, if the head allows, the clitoris will follow. We encourage women to experiment with a range of methods to achieve sexual arousal, and vary them, whether with a partner or without. Sometimes the emotional/romantic pleasure experienced during a shared encounter can be as powerful as the physical pleasure experienced from a vibrator, and vice versa.

Am I Supposed to Be an Actress?

Jane, a successful professional woman in her early thirties, sat in our office, clearly agitated. As her hands gripped the sides of the armchair, she explained that she had come to seek our counsel after a particularly disturbing appointment with the couple's therapist she and her husband had been seeing for the past several months. The subject of sex had come up and Jane's husband said that he did not feel Jane was "responsive" enough in bed. This came to Jane as a surprise, given that she had always been able to have orgasms with her husband. Responding to her husband's comment, Jane explained that the (male) therapist told her that her "problem" was her quiet demeanor during sexual arousal. "You do not ooh and aah during the act," he told her. "You do not talk dirty . . . You do not vocalize, you do not scream in ecstasy."

Jane told us she felt outraged and confused. "Am I the only woman who does not ooh and aah?" she asked. "How dare he say this to me? Am I supposed to be an actress or am I supposed to be me?"

Unfortunately, Jane's therapist is not alone in adhering to a male-centric, media-driven perception of what a woman's orgasm is "supposed to sound like." We've all seen the movies where the leading man abruptly overcomes his female counterpart, who, amid much hair-grabbing and back-scratching, is brought to a loud, thundering climax within moments of penetration. Beyond presenting unrealistic ideals of physical and sexual perfection, these media-induced fantasies find their way into many men's and women's subconscious, limiting our ability to fully enjoy the uniqueness of our own sexual experiences.

The truth is we all have our own individual sexual styles. When it comes to orgasm, some women are quiet while others are loud; some talk "dirty" while others prefer to speak more romantically; some sigh while others moan; some like to close their eyes while others prefer to look at their partners. While there should be clear communication to ensure that both partners are satisfied, there should be no mandating of vocalization—or of anything else—during sexual intimacy. It is a time of freedom of expression, of being yourself and enjoying the moment *in a way that feels right for you.*

Should I Use a Lubricant?

In short: yes, unless you are wet enough to engage sexually without any chafing, "hot spots," or irritation. Feeling that you're naturally lubricated enough—or your partner telling you that you're lubricated enough—does not necessarily mean you are sufficiently lubricated for comfortable penetration and thrusting. Using a lubricant is especially important if you're having repeated sexual encounters within a short period of time or if intercourse with your partner tends to last long enough that you begin to experience irritation. This also applies to prolonged use of sexual toys, whether clitoral or vaginal, such as a dildo inserted into the vagina.

It's also important to remember that a woman's need for lubrication will vary at different points in her life. A woman in her twenties or thirties, for example, may require less lubrication than a woman going through menopause or a woman who has undergone medical treatment for cancer or other medical conditions.

While some may be resistant to using a lubricant ("it's messy," "I don't like the way it smells," "shouldn't my own lubrication be enough?" "my partner doesn't like it,") we encourage you to experiment until you find one that works for you. Let yourself explore through a process of trial and error.

Shop around for the lubricant you like and, of course, make sure that it does not react with your skin. Water-based and sugar-free formulas are often preferred to minimize genital irritation. We also recommend looking for a lubricant with a convenient dispenser, which will simplify application and make you more likely to use it. However, we advise staying away from mint flavors, as well as any formulas with extra additives, as they tend to irritate the vulva.

You might consider, for example, using flavored lubricants for oral sex. Why, you ask?

- For fun—who wants boring sex?
- For variety—experiment with different flavors.
- For additional clitoral lubrication.
- To mask genital smell—not everyone cares for "natural odors."

'Killing' an Orgasm

How can you kill an orgasm, you ask? Very easily. Take the case of Shauna, who came to us with the complaint that she just couldn't seem to have orgasms anymore. Married to her high school sweetheart, Shauna and her husband both worked full-time while raising two energetic toddlers. "It's hard enough getting any time alone with my husband at all," she told us. "We're both so tired by the end of the day, that we crash the minute our heads hit the pillow. On the rare occasions when we do manage to find time to be intimate, it's hard for me to really get into it. Lately, I've been having trouble climaxing, which is a problem I never had before."

Shauna was concerned that her difficulty reaching orgasm might be medical in nature, but as she spoke, it became clear that her problem was not rooted in any physical causes. "Even while Steve and I are in the middle of being sexual, all I can think about is, what if one of our kids wakes up? Even when I know they're sound asleep, I can't help worrying that they might hear us—or worse, that they'll walk in. I never liked the idea of putting a lock on our bedroom door, but now I wonder . . ."

Shauna's predicament is not unusual. Ideally, sexual intimacy requires us to take a break from the endless "to-do" lists running through our brains and instead focus on the physical and emotional pleasure of physical closeness. In this scenario, we let go and give ourselves over to the pleasurable sensations at hand—kind of like eating the best chocolate dessert ever and 'being in the zone' body and mind. But for most women, our minds play the role of filter during sexual intimacy, and any stray thought or the faintest worry has the potential to kill our pleasure. And it's not only the "big" worries about family, work, or money, but anything that happens to be on our minds—from who's going to do the grocery shopping to whether or not to shower before getting intimate. Yes, the clitoris is the primary female sexual organ, but a woman's sexuality is filtered through her mind and emotions.

Things that may inhibit arousal and kill orgasm include:

- **A preoccupied mind.** The inability to stop thinking about all you have to do: the dishes in the sink, the project due at work tomorrow . . .
- **A worried mind.** Will the kids walk in? Will my parents hear us? Should I answer the phone? Will my roommate come home sooner than expected?
- **A self-conscious mind.** Will my partner notice my stretch marks/cellulite/the fact that I've put on weight? Am I clean enough down there? What if he doesn't like how I smell? Am I as good in bed as his last girlfriend?
- **Relationship issues.** Feeling emotionally or physically unsafe; This isn't what I want; I'm doing it to please my partner; sexual boredom.
- **Communication fears and concerns.** I don't know how to tell my partner how I like to be touched. It takes me longer to "get there" and I feel bad for him. Maybe I should just fake it and get it over with???

Of course, even in the healthiest of sexual relationships, we may "lose it" for one of the above reasons or perhaps for no reason at all. Furthermore, not all women will necessarily reach orgasm every time they're aroused, and at times, may tell their partner they prefer something else, like a back rub or foot massage. However, if this is something that's happening on a regular basis, it might be beneficial to think about whether any of the above descriptions apply to you.

While some women may tell themselves, "it's no big deal," and others simply become despairing, it's important to remember that by allowing your orgasms to be killed on a regular basis, you run the risk of developing a pattern, which affects both you and your partner. Unfortunately, it is easy for many women to forgo their own sexual satisfaction, particularly in the context of a long-term relationship. For this reason, we like to remind women that it's easier to prevent a habit from forming than trying to undo an entrenched dynamic years down the road.

The first step in overcoming this pattern is to become aware of the thoughts or concerns that may be getting in the way of your orgasm. The second step is learning how to create a private space for yourself and your partner—no matter how busy you are, no matter what else is happening in your life. We've named this space "The Intimate Zone."

The Intimate Zone

The intimate zone is what we call that special connection a couple shares that cannot be shared with anyone else. Of course, there is the sexual component of this connection, but it is not only sexual. The intimate zone implies a time and place shared with your partner where you can be whoever and whatever you want. It's a space where you feel free to exchange and explore in a way that you wouldn't even with the closest of friends. Indeed, without such a space, the couple is, in fact, no more than friends, living together "like brother and sister," as some of our patients have put it.

The intimate zone stands apart from the rest of our everyday lives—a mindset as much as a specific place, where work and kids and bills do not exist. It's a place where we can focus less on *doing*, and more on *being*. We may talk, laugh, cuddle, touch, listen, or simply breathe. Every couple's intimate zone is unique to them—the point is a safe space devoted to being together.

It's important to remember that an intimate zone doesn't just happen—it has to be created. One woman we know, who was in a loving and happy relationship, explained to us that she and her husband scheduled specific times throughout the week to be together. Whether they spent that time in bed or going for a walk in the park, their rule remained the same: no "business" talk, with business being anything from mortgage payments to how the kids were doing in school, to the in-laws' upcoming visit. They even devised an arrangement whereby if one of them happened to mention a "business" matter during one of their set-aside times, he or she would owe the other $20!

Although this particular approach may not work for everyone, the point is a crucial one: If we want our relationships to thrive, we need to actively carve out time to focus on them—without distractions. That may mean turning off or putting away electronic devices, hiring a babysitter for a couple of hours, or putting a lock on the bedroom door.

Here are some other tips:

- Create a relaxing environment. Light candles, play music . . .
- Take turns scheduling something special: an activity, a date, a vacation, etc.
- Let humor in. Talk about your dreams, explore new mutual interests . . .
- Make sex fun; it does not have to be serious! Also, experiment. Step out of your comfort zone and try different positions. Introduce vibrators/powered toys.
- Let fantasy in. Share your fantasies with your partner, sexual or otherwise. Invite him or her to do the same.
- Be honest. Don't be afraid to say what you want—or what you don't want.

Giving yourself permission to enjoy such an intimate space benefits not just your relationship, but you as an individual. We all need a place where we can relax and be ourselves. Don't you deserve it?

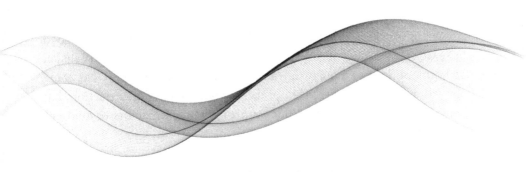

Chapter Six

Your Body, Your Relationship

Negotiating Sexual Compatibility

I n the search for a partner, we assess potential mates against an endless list of qualifications—everything from physical attraction to family background to religious affiliation to education level and career goals to whether or not we like the same music or share a love of sports. It should go without saying that a person's sexual style and preferences are critical considerations in determining whether a relationship will work. It is important to remember that there are no rights and wrongs when it comes to sharing a healthy, pleasurable sexual relationship with another person. As long as the activity is safe and consensual, we encourage women to have fun and experiment. As we like to tell our patients, if they and their partner are both into it, why not?

However, all too often, women feel hesitant, embarrassed, or apprehensive about taking an honest look at whether we and our partners are sexually sympatico. Typically this is because we are less comfortable prioritizing the sexual aspects of the relationship, often deferring to our partners' inclinations or desires instead. While this may seem like the "safer" or "easier" route initially, it inevitably lays the groundwork for problems down the road. It is worth noting that this may be challenging for women raised in more traditional cultures that prohibit any contact or exploration outside of marriage, putting pressure on women to transition "overnight" into sexual compatibility.

When we speak of sexual compatibility—of two people being a "good fit"—we are speaking, of course, about much more than genital size, shape, or hormone levels (though those may be important as well). The most obvious question is whether or not there is mutual physical attraction, but sexual compatibility also depends on a wide range of factors beyond our bodies' hardwiring:

- What are our sexual expectations of our partner?
- Do we hope the sexual arena will "solve" other problems in the relationship?
- How do we see ourselves and our own bodies?
- Do we know how to ask for what we need or desire?
- Is there passion?
- Are we committed to working on our sexual connection, and able to communicate effectively and respectfully about it?
- Do we have a shared view on contraception and on whether or not we want to have children?
- Are there religious differences that may affect the sexual relationship?
- Does one's prior sexual experience negatively affect the relationship?
- Is one partner more interested in sex than the other, or less? Or interested in different kinds of sexual experiences?
- Is our sex life safe and consensual, or is it forced? Demanded?

Part of compatibility entails synching up our rhythm of arousal with our partner's. Sometimes, the man may please the woman before engaging in intercourse, while some couples may reverse the rotation, and others may prioritize climaxing simultaneously. (This applies to lesbian couples as well.) It is the responsibility of both partners to work together not only to find the sexual activities that they both enjoy, but also to learn how to align their rhythms in a way that feels comfortable and satisfying for both of them.

In this chapter, we will examine both the physical and emotional challenges to sexual intimacy that we see most frequently in our practice. As we'll discuss, some incompatibilities are resolvable, while others may not be. If two people are willing and open, however, adjustments and compromises can usually be made to everyone's satisfaction. *Ultimately, sexual* compatibility depends upon knowing what your needs and wants are and being willing to express them. It's about allowing yourself to be vulnerable in front of another person. It's about learning, over time, how to both give and receive.

Sexual Templates: Hers and His

One of our starting points for understanding human sexuality is acknowledging the fundamental differences that exist between men and women when it comes to sex, which we refer to as the "sexual template."[5] Generally speaking, women thrive on affection—talking, hugging, kissing, and sharing feelings. Men, on the other hand, typically feel most appreciated through the sexual act itself. For a woman, sexual arousal necessitates shutting down the thinking/preoccupied/worried brain; for a man, sexual arousal itself can quiet any potential anxieties. To put it another way, a woman's sexual feelings are filtered through her mind, while a man's sexual feelings (temporarily) shut down his mind.

Another important contrast between the male and female sexual template has to do with the relationships we have with our own genitals. From a young age, men are intimately aware of their penis and its bodily functions of urination and pleasure, making it easier for them, as they mature, to transition into sexual activity. However, this is not the case for women: the vagina is invisible and is not involved in elimination, thus rendering it "mysterious." The clitoris is similarly hidden within the folds of the vulva, unless discovered through exploration. Furthermore, religious, cultural and societal prohibitions often discourage women from exploring and learning about their genitals. It is not unusual for us to meet grown women who lack a basic vocabulary to discuss sexuality and are unaware of the clitoris and its role in sexual pleasure.

Now, before we go any further, let us acknowledge that these are obviously generalizations. Sexually speaking, we will not respond to the same stimuli in the same way every time; many men cherish affection, and enjoy both giving and receiving it, but if the relationship does not include some form of sexual connection, they will likely feel incomplete. Likewise, we certainly don't

---

5. In lesbian relationships, the psychosexual dynamics will reflect their shared sexual template.

mean to imply that women can't value and enjoy sex—of course they can and they do. Still, our clinical observations have shown they can delay sexual engagement or gratification for hours, days, or in some cases years on end, provided there is some form of intimate affection in their lives. For women, sexual engagement is a choice, not necessarily a need.

While the differences between female and male sexual templates are undoubtedly influenced by cultural, religious, even socioeconomic factors, their origins are rooted in biology. Evolutionarily speaking, females seek sex (mating) for reproductive purposes only, a function that naturally diminishes with age. Genetically, males are equipped with a vivid sexual imagination that recruits all five senses and does not lessen over time, so as to increase the odds of procreation and curb natural attrition. That is why a man can easily get turned on at the sight of a naked woman, while a woman is more likely to get turned on by a thoughtful gesture, great conversation, or a day of romantic relaxation.

As women, our sexual feelings will almost always reflect our feelings about the relationship. We need to feel appreciated and valued as people in order to be sexually interested. At the very least, we want to feel like our partner is looking out for us, and taking our needs into consideration. As one of our patients memorably put it, "If my husband doesn't take out the garbage, there's no way I can find him sexy."

While the contrasts in the male and female sexual template will present themselves differently for every couple, the following are the most common:

- **Variety.** Men, animated by an active sexual imagination, want a dynamic sexual variety—whether in positions, locations, activities, or vocalization—all geared toward increased arousal.
- *Foreplay/Afterplay.* Women typically crave more time spent kissing and touching, whether it's before, during, after, or instead of intercourse. In other words, it's more about affection and romance than stimulation of one's "hardware." Nevertheless, a woman's sexual arousal will require clitoral stimulation, either direct or indirect.
- **Timing.** Women tend not to be into "quickies" (when time is pressed, before the kids come back, when company is staying over, etc.), which require an instant shutting down of the thinking mind to allow for a fast arousal, whereas men are quite good

at it, because of their above-mentioned efficient arousability. So the timing of sexual engagement may need to be negotiated. In addition, it's not unusual for a man to want sex in the morning, when his hormone levels are at their peak, while a woman's mind is preoccupied with the day ahead: getting ready for work, making sure the kids are ready for school, etc. Other timing consideration may include frequency of sexual engagement (most men would love it as often as possible even if their bodies may not be up for it), intimacy during menstruation, pregnancy, or in the midst of a disagreement or other relationship struggles.

- **Relaxation.** In general, women need to feel relaxed in order to have sex, while for men, sex itself is a tool for relaxation.

- **Connection.** The female sexual template needs communication and affection to trigger arousal, whereas for a man, the act itself is a vehicle to express feelings. In other words, a woman's sexual satisfaction is measured by the quality of her connection with her partner.

- **Duration of arousal.** Men typically seek to prolong their arousal as long as possible, whether during outercourse or intercourse, and they can do it quite well. However, such efforts can exceed women's physical and/or emotional tolerance. When sexual activity is taking longer than a woman desires, she should listen to her body and let her partner know if she's getting tired or uncomfortable, and/or take a break to apply additional lubrication if necessary.

- **Age/life-cycle.** A woman is typically more sexually active during her child-bearing years, and less so as she gets older. (See Chapter 8 for more on sexuality after menopause.) In addition, the longer a woman has been in a relationship, the less sexually excited she will be, unless she and her partner make specific efforts to keep their sexual relationship alive and exciting. Indeed, it's not unusual for women in long-term relationships to report feeling bored with their sexual relationships, since "I know all his moves." Men, on the other hand, maintain a consistently active sexual interest regardless of age.

Does Size Matter?

While as a rule, the male and female bodies are built for intercourse, there are times when size matters.

The penis has two dimensions: length and girth (thickness).

- The length will fit in as deep as the vaginal canal will allow. In most cases, the penis will fit completely, while in other cases (i.e., a super long penis, an unusually short vagina, or a surgically-shortened vagina), the base of the shaft may remain outside. Some positions may afford greater vaginal depth, so it is worth experimenting.
- Girth poses a problem because a thicker-than-average penis will challenge the vaginal opening, sometimes leading to painful tearing of the vaginal tissue. In rare cases, a very thick penis (yes, they do exist) may make vaginal intercourse impossible altogether.

Not long ago we saw a woman in our office complaining she was unable to have intercourse with her husband because of his size.

"He feels too big to fit inside my vagina," she told us matter-of-factly. "When we try, I feel that I am being torn from the inside—and my vaginal opening will often bleed. We keep trying, but he cannot get inside me for normal intercourse."

She told us that her husband had admitted that a previous partner had also told him he was bigger than average, but that, somehow, they still managed to have "a regular sex life."

"I know it's my fault," she told us. "My vagina's just too small. To tell you the truth, I've been looking into undergoing surgery to expand my vagina."

We explained that the vagina is rarely too small in structure. However, when a woman is tense, nervous, or afraid, her vagina may seem smaller or tighter; but otherwise, it is able to accommodate an average to slightly thicker than average penis. We added that a woman should never blame herself—or allow herself to be blamed—for being "too small." (Nor should she accept a diagnosis of vaginismus or dyspareunia before a medical professional has ascertained that her partner's penis is of functional girth.)

Having examined her and reaffirmed that her "small vagina" is actually perfectly normal in size, we counseled her to rethink the option of surgical vaginal expansion, which unnecessarily alters a woman's anatomy and medicalizes her sexuality, encouraging her to view her own body as the problem. We reminded her that she has no reason to feel that she has "failed," nor any cause to believe that she is inadequate in any way.

That said, we recommended gently stretching the vaginal opening prior to intercourse with a comparably sized dilator or dildo—and, of course, plenty of lubricant. We also suggested that she and her husband undergo a series of sexual counseling sessions, not only to learn how to better facilitate partial or complete intercourse, but also how to enjoy each other sexually in a variety of ways.

A final note on size: It is a common misconception that a man or woman's genitals corresponds to their physical stature. Nothing could be further from the truth. A person's height or body type has no bearing whatsoever on genital size. A tall man may have a small penis, and vice versa. The same applies to women and the size of their vaginas.

Medical Matters

Some forms of sexual incompatibility are medical in origin—though as we will see, the positive resolution of even these challenges will depend on a willingness on the part of each partner to assert clear and open communication about how they are feeling, both physically and emotionally. Often, women exhibit more reticence in this regard than men.

Not long ago, we saw a fifty-year-old woman named Janine in our office. Janine reported that intercourse with her husband had been physically uncomfortable for the last twenty years of their twenty-two-year marriage. As a result of this long-term discomfort, she had developed chronic yeast- and urinary tract infections. Over the years, she had seen countless doctors and specialists, none of whom were able to determine the source of her problem.

We promptly took a thorough medical and emotional history, during which Janine revealed that her husband suffered from symptoms we recognized as Peyronie's disease. Peyronie's disease, a condition of uncertain cause, is characterized by the formation of a plaque or hard lump on the penis, causing it to bend during erection. A plaque on the top of the shaft (most common) causes the penis to bend upward; a plaque on the underside causes it to bend downward. In some cases, the plaque develops on both top and bottom, leading to indentation and shortening of the penis. Depending on the severity of the condition, the bend in the penis may make sexual intercourse difficult, or even impossible. And if he is able to penetrate the vagina, the action of thrusting (the penis motion during intercourse) by a bent penis may cause discomfort to the woman, often to the point of friction irritation.

In Janine's case, it was clear to us that it was her husband's condition that was the cause of her painful intercourse and chronic infections—a connection that had not previously been made. Neither Janine nor her husband had considered the possibility that the source of the problem lay with him—not an uncommon dynamic for couples when issues of sexual incompatibility arise. Like Janine, many women are quick to assume that they are the "problematic" ones. It is important for women to realize that this is simply not the case; men may have physical issues with their penises that should be explored. Peyronie's disease is just one example; in other cases, a man may be dealing with erectile dysfunction, premature ejaculation, or surgical procedures that result in the penis being altered, enlarged, or extremely sensitive.

Men will always be protective of their penis's health while women are often reluctant advocates for their vagina and clitoris, to the detriment of themselves and their relationships. We explained to Janine that in order to protect her health, intercourse was not advisable. Janine initially became distraught, not wanting to upset her husband or hurt his feelings. Knowing this would be a highly charged discussion, we nevertheless encouraged her and her husband to seek adjustments, modifications, and alternate forms of sexual satisfaction from the Sexual Menu. In addition, we recommended considering sexual counseling if further intervention is needed.

Why Can't a Hug be Just a Hug? Conflict, Communication, and Make-Up Sex

Diana was a recently married woman in her mid-twenties who came to see us for sexual counseling. The problem, as she described it, was that she and her husband of three years rarely had sex. The more they did not have sex, she explained, the more they argued, and the more they argued, the less she wanted to have sex. Diana was finishing graduate school, so money was tight, and her husband was under a great deal of pressure trying to prove himself at a new job. In the meantime, their relationship was deteriorating rapidly. Diana understood that she and her husband were caught in a vicious cycle, and that they would need help getting out of it.

Part of the problem, Diana explained, was not even the arguments themselves, but what happened afterward. Typically after a fight, Diana would go to their bedroom and lie down, waiting for her husband to come in and apologize. But rather than saying he was sorry, or attempting to see things from her perspective, he often wanted to resolve things by becoming sexually intimate. "Sometimes, after we've been arguing, he'll come over and give me a hug. And I'll think, 'Oh, that's really sweet.' But then, he'll start pressing against me and his hands start going to undo my bra, and I think, 'Is he crazy? I'm way too upset to even consider sex right now.' Then he ends up feeling rejected, which turns into another fight. I don't understand why he always has to take it in that direction. Why can't a hug just be a hug?"

Indeed, this question—and its countless variations—is among the most common we hear. When it comes to "make-up sex," our clinical observations suggest a clear difference between the genders. And here lies another key distinction between the male and female sexual templates: **While a man will seek sexual encounter as a tool for resolution of conflict, a woman will typically only enter a sexual encounter once the conflict has been resolved.**

We shared with Diana that simply acknowledging and making room for such differences might help break the cycle of arguments over this persistent flashpoint of sexual incompatibility. We recommended that in a quiet moment, Diana discuss with her husband their respective approaches to resolving conflict, and what a meaningful "make-up" might look like for each of them, without blaming or judging the other person's preference.

Once Diana's husband became aware of how his wife's needs differed from his own, he agreed not to initiate sexual contact after they'd been fighting. Instead, with the help of a therapist, they learned how to improve their communication both during and after conflicts and to seek out opportunities for sexual closeness that were amenable to both of them, which would begin with allocating time to simply "be" together without any sexual expectations.

I'm Just Not Interested: the Busy Mind

Complaints of sexual boredom are also common in our practice. They are so common, in fact, that some women take it for granted, accepting their disinterest as a way of life. We urge women not to settle for the status quo, but rather to explore the underlying causes so that they can enjoy the kind of sexual closeness they deserve.

A busy mother of two and high school English teacher, Iris made an appointment to see us because she was concerned she might be experiencing a serious medical problem. "I have no libido whatsoever," Iris told us. "My husband complains constantly that we never have sex." In her mid-thirties, Iris and her husband had been married for ten years. In the early years of their relationship, she explained, they'd enjoyed an active sex life. "I still love my husband," she told us. "But if you would have told me ten years ago that Marc and I never have sex anymore, I wouldn't have believed you."

When we asked Iris what had changed, she laughed. "Well, for one thing, I hardly ever have a moment to myself, let alone time alone with Marc. In the mornings, I'm busy getting my daughters ready for school, or finishing last-minute lesson plans. After teaching all day, I pick up the girls from school, help them with their homework, make dinner, and try to catch up on the laundry. Once the girls have gone to bed, is the first chance I get to sit down and grade my students' papers. I'm often up past 10 or 11 pm, because that's simply the only time I can get the work done."

Concerned that her ongoing fatigue and low sex drive might be symptoms of an illness, Iris had made an appointment with her general practitioner, who, to her surprise, reported her to be in good health. Listening to Iris speak, it was clear to us that she was not suffering from some mysterious medical affliction, nor was she suffering from a "low sex drive" per se. Instead, her problem seemed to be that she did not have the time and space necessary to **shut off her mind**.

This is, of course, perfectly understandable. As women, we often do double-duty as caregivers and breadwinners, our days and nights filled with unfinished projects, looming deadlines, or piles of papers to grade. If we experience a lack of interest in sexual activity, it is vital that we not rush to medicalize our feelings, but first consider them in the context of the rest of our lives. Over and over, our clinical experience has shown that for most women, the cause of a so-called low libido is more likely to be found in the mind than in the body.

As we spoke more with Iris in subsequent sessions, it became apparent that what she and her husband needed most was to learn how to carve out space dedicated exclusively to their relationship—sexual and otherwise—amidst their busy lives. At our suggestion, they decided to set aside one night during the week, or one afternoon during the weekend, just for them. The focus, we explained, should be the enjoyment of uninterrupted time together, investing in "their intimate zone." This meant hiring a babysitter or arranging play dates for their daughters. It also meant no phone, no laptop, no iPad, and no grading papers. Once she and her husband learned how to create a private, intimate space for themselves, no matter how busy things were, Iris gradually felt the return of her sexual interest. Not only did she come to feel better about her marriage, the resurgence of her sexual identity helped Iris to feel better about herself and life in general.

As women, it is not unusual for our sexual relationships to take a back seat when we are feeling overwhelmed by life's demands. In other cases, it is not necessarily the busy-ness of work, partnership, or parenthood that leaves us feeling sexually bored and disinterested, but simply the passage of time.

I'm Just Not Interested: Sexual Boredom

Jacqueline was another woman who came to our office complaining of low sex drive. A stay at home mom with three young children, she had been with her husband, Paul, since their first year of college. Jacqueline was able to recall the passionate late nights with Paul in her dorm room, but those were now a thing of the distant past, she told us. As they had kids, bought a house—"all the things I'd dreamed of" —the sexual excitement in their relationship disappeared. "It's because of me," Jacqueline told us. "Paul is a wonderful husband and I love him. But for a while now, it feels more like I'm just living with a roommate. He's still interested in me, but it's like that part of me just died."

Even on those occasions when they would plan a "date night," she confessed, she would often find a way to get out of it. "At 10 a.m., I'd be looking forward to spending time with Paul later that night. But by 4 p.m., the house is a mess and the kids are crabby and dinner's not made. By the time Paul gets home, and we eat dinner and give the kids baths, I'm just too tired. It really hurts Paul's feelings. I keep telling him it's not about him, but I think that makes him feel even worse."

Jacqueline's experience highlights yet again the differences between the female and male sexual templates. It is not uncommon, once a relationship is established and of long standing, for a woman's excitement about the sexual aspect of the relationship to diminish or even disappear. When a woman has been with her partner for years (or even decades), it can become easy for her to forgo sexual connection—there's certainly no rush, and she typically has a thousand other things on her plate that need her attention. While, as women, we may enjoy our orgasms, we may find, with the passage of the years, that we can live without them, or self masturbate to orgasm without being with a partner. It's not unusual for women in well-established partnerships to find that a foot massage or back rub is more satisfying than a full-fledged sexual encounter. Biologically speaking, it is "natural" for a woman to lose sexual interest over time. But while this course of events may be natural, it is not inevitable.

In our practice, we encourage women not to allow themselves to become entrenched in their own disinterest. A long-term partnership requires an ongoing maintenance of the sexual connection, without which the relationship is not really a partnership, but a friendship, or for some, merely a shared living arrangement. By avoiding intimacy on a regular basis, a woman runs the risk of developing a pattern, which can quickly become the status quo. Not only does this threaten the happiness and viability of the relationship, it also robs a woman of the opportunity to be close to another person in the most intimate sense.

While we recommend counseling with a licensed therapist to help work through the deeper issues that may be underlying sexual disinterest, we have seen many cases in which making a conscious decision to invest in the Intimate Zone has had a significant impact not only on the relationship, but on the individuals' personal sense of wellbeing. Planning a romantic getaway (even if only for one night!), surprising your partner with a thoughtful, unexpected gesture, or even just meeting for coffee or lunch in the middle of a busy day are small steps that can help reignite feelings of closeness. We never tire of reminding our patients that sexual interest is not something that happens by itself—like anything else of value, it needs to be cultivated.

I've Lost My Libido

There are countless reasons why a woman may develop a disinterest in sex. This is rarely the result of any particular pathology, and more likely caused by one or more of the following:

▸ Sexual boredom.
▸ Underlying tensions or outright dislike of one's partner.
▸ The inability to shut down one's mind (in some cases exacerbated by generalized anxiety disorder or obsessive compulsive disorder).
▸ Poor body image or other psychological inhibitions.
▸ Physical fatigue.
▸ Fear of pain.
▸ Fear of loss of control.
▸ Concern about sexually transmitted infection (STI) or pregnancy.
▸ Religious demands or expectations (from one's partner, family, or both).
▸ The inability to say "no," to speak up preferences, to choose. if one wants to engage sexually or to be left alone.
▸ Certain prescription medications.
▸ A partner's infidelity.
▸ Negative or traumatic sexual experiences from the past.

Always the Giver: the Danger of 'Absenting' Ourselves

Because many of us are socialized from girlhood "not to touch down there" or that our sexuality must be "saved" for marriage, it can be difficult for us to know what we like in the first place. Bring a partner into the mix and it can get even more complicated. How can we tell our partners how they can satisfy us when we don't know ourselves? Rather than take the time to educate ourselves about our bodies and desires, it can be all too easy for many of us to simply become the "givers" in our sexual relationships. So often the cases we see in our office are not ones of sexual incompatibility per se, but instances in which a woman has opted to absent herself—sexually, emotionally, or both.

When Maureen, a woman in her mid-forties, came to see us at our offices she told us plainly that she was there out of desperation. In her mid-forties with three teenage children, Maureen had been married for seventeen years in a relationship she described as "basically happy." But now her husband was saying that after years of being sexually unsatisfied, he wanted a divorce.

Growing up in a strict Catholic family, Maureen had been taught both at school and at home that her "private parts were dirty." Only through the sacrament of marriage, she was taught, could the sex act be redeemed. When Maureen met her future husband when they were both counselors at a Catholic summer camp, she explained, "We knew there was no question we would wait until we were married."

While Maureen and her husband had no problem having intercourse, she was never able to really enjoy it, nor any other form of sexual closeness. For one thing, Maureen explained, she'd maintained a life-long aversion to having her genitals touched in any way. "In the beginning of our marriage, my husband wanted me to let him touch my vagina or even perform oral sex on me, but I would never let him. I knew he was disappointed, so I tried to make up for it by always being the giver. I had no problem giving him oral sex or having intercourse, even though, I can't say I ever really enjoyed either.

"To be honest, I never really thought there was much of a problem until the last few years when my husband started saying that he wanted 'more.' Now he says he doesn't want to stay in the relationship because there's not enough passion, whatever that means. He keeps saying, 'I want a participating partner,' but I just don't know if I can give him what he wants."

Eventually, it became clear that sadly, Maureen was right. By the time she came to see us, her husband had already made up his mind. He'd already been patient enough, he claimed, and after nearly twenty years of unfulfilling sex, he'd lost any hope that things would improve. It was too late for her marriage to be salvaged, but through a series of sexual counseling sessions, she was able to gain a deeper understanding of herself. While a part of her wished she had managed to seek help years earlier, she also felt confident that at this point in her life she knew herself better that she ever had before.

Moving Past Conflicts

When a relationship is stuck in a place of conflict, it can be hard to see our way out of it. Particularly in the sexual arena, it can be easier to pretend the problem doesn't exist, or think that, magically, the situation will somehow improve on its own. While maintaining the status quo and "hoping" things will get better may seem easier in the short run, it deprives us of the opportunity to get to know ourselves and our partners better and to open up meaningful channels of communication and sexual fulfillment.

Whether you're dealing with a longstanding sexual conflict, or simply disappointed by the quality of closeness in your sexual relationship, acknowledging your feelings— even if it's only to yourself—is an important first step. From there, you will need to decide how (and if) to broach the topic with your partner and which resources to consider. Typically, facing a sexual conflict requires a three-pronged approach that takes into account our physical, sexual, *and* mental well-being.

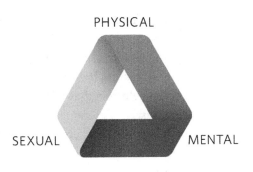

Regardless of your age, or how long you've been "tolerating" the situation, you may want to consider some of the following:

- **Body awareness.** As mentioned earlier in this chapter, we may lack a basic understanding of our bodies and how they function, particularly when it comes to our genitals. We never tire of reminding our patients that knowledge is power. We believe that in order to have a truly satisfying sexual relationship, a woman needs to become an expert on her own body.
- **Sex education.** Doing our homework, whether by reading books, seeking information online, or undergoing sexual counseling,

can help expand our knowledge and understanding of how to get the most out of our sexual relationships. It can also help to provide us with the language to discuss sensitive topics.

- **Self esteem.** Self-esteem issues are often the underlying cause of sexual dysfunction. Getting to the root of self-esteem issues with the help of a mental health professional can have a significant impact not only on one's sex life, but on one's life as a whole.

- **Mental health.** Sometimes our sexual relationships are impacted by undiagnosed or untreated disorders such as anxiety, panic, depression, and obsessive-compulsive disorder. In such cases, it is unlikely that our sexual relationship will improve until we address the underlying problem.

- **Partner's sexuality.** In some cases, sexual conflict or incompatibility can be traced directly to a partner's sexual health, making it vital that he or she seek necessary medical/mental treatment as well.

- **Relationship issues.** As we've said before, the sexual relationship serves as a mirror of a relationship's overall health. If there are ongoing tensions, resentments, or disagreements that are not being addressed, they will always impact the sexual connection. Seeking help together with one's partner can be vital in such situations.

- **Family pressure.** Pressure to live the way our parents expect us to, adhere to religious traditions, or procreate on demand can all sour the sexual relationship. Unsolicited advice and intrusions from our families, and especially from our in-laws, can impact the sexual relationship, as we find ourselves "shutting down" or using disinterest as a weapon to punish our partners.

To Tell or Not to Tell? Learning What You Want and How to Ask For It

So often we hear women say, "I want to talk to my partner, but I don't know how," or "I try to talk to him but he doesn't listen." Sometimes, it can seem easier to keep one's feelings to oneself rather than face the frustration of not being heard—particularly when it comes to the sensitive subject of sex. It's not uncommon for us to see patients grappling with the question of whether or not to share their experiences with their partners, or how to overcome shyness or embarrassment discussing such intimate topics—especially if they've never done so before.

While men are typically quite clear about their sexual likes and dislikes, women are often hesitant to speak their minds, opting instead to go through the motions and suffer in silence and/or develop chronic disinterest. It is not unusual for women to wonder if they should express to their partner truths like

- Intercourse is not arousing.
- Intercourse is painful.
- I need lubrication for comfortable intercourse.
- I want him to wear a condom.
- I want to discuss his/her testing for sexually transmitted infections.
- I prefer a different sexual position.
- I need more foreplay.
- I want to be intimate, but don't want to have intercourse.
- As much as he tries, I still can't reach orgasm.
- It takes me so long to get aroused that I am worried partner is getting impatient or annoyed with me.
- His efforts to arouse me are doing nothing for me.
- I have never had intercourse.
- I am nervous about pain when resuming sexual activity after childbirth, or because of menopause, vaginismus, surgery, cancer treatment, etc.
- I just don't feel like it today.

If you're reading this book, you probably know that our answer to all of these questions is a resounding YES. Barring extreme situations where a woman fears for her life or safety, when debating whether to tell or not to tell, we will always advocate for sharing with one's partner. The fact is that without communication, there is no relationship—just two people coexisting in parallel lives.

Across all areas of life—whether in business, friendship, or family relationships— the purpose of communication is for two people to get to know each other, exchange preferences, and identify areas of disagreement or conflict. These components are especially crucial in a sexual relationship, which depends upon negotiation, adjustment, and compromise. Despite what the media might tell us, this is not a sign of a relationship's weakness, but of its strength.

And yet, the question remains: How do we begin talking to our partners about our most personal (and for some of us, most shameful) needs, wants, and desires? The first rule is to be honest. Our partners cannot read our minds, nor is it their job to do so. It is our responsibility to let our partners know what we like, what we don't like, what turns us on and what doesn't.

We encourage women to take the time to examine their hesitancies or inhibitions. It can be helpful to sit down, with pen and paper if necessary, and take an inventory of one's sexual relationship. Are you typically satisfied after a sexual encounter? Do you feel like something's missing but are afraid to bring it up? Are there fantasies that you are keeping from your partner? Many of our patients have found it worthwhile to simply ask themselves, what do I really want from my sexual relationship? How do I want to be talked to? How do I want to be touched?

It bears repeating: If you don't tell your partner, he or she won't know. And if he or she doesn't know, how can the situation improve? As women, we need to remember that we have the right to express our desires—even if we are afraid our partners may be insulted or hurt by the feedback. While some of us may feel that we're risking the stability of our relationships by communicating openly, it is worth asking ourselves why we are choosing to prioritize our partners' feelings over our own.

It's also helpful to remember that communication need not be verbal only. We encourage our patients to use any means at their disposal—a word, a gesture, a letter, even a text message—to share with their partners. While some of us will be comfortable inviting our partners to sit down for a frank, in-depth discussion, others of us may simply choose to take our partner's hand and show him what we want.

Why Suffer in Silence?

Unfortunately, women tend to keep their feelings to themselves and act as sexual subservients instead of equal partners. What keeps a woman from speaking up and making her needs known? Societal, cultural, and religious influences play a key role in complicated and overlapping ways that impact an already-fragile emotional state. Whatever the ultimate cause, the resulting feelings of shame and confusion often end up deeply embedded in women's psyches.

- Low self-esteem: "I don't deserve any better."
- Feeling stuck: "It is my job and duty to satisfy my husband's sexual needs . . ."
- Feelings of isolation: "I am the only one struggling, so I may as well keep quiet."
- Fear of being alone: "If I speak up, my partner will leave me."
- Family and/or community pressure: "In my culture, women submit. Speaking up will only lead to negative repercussions."

When it comes to sexual activity of any kind, no one deserves to feel helpless, hopeless, or forced-upon. *It should always be the woman's choice whether, and in what form, she wants to engage sexually, which, sadly, is not yet an available option to all women worldwide.*

Intimacy and Honesty

We like to remind all women that **there is no intimacy without honesty.**

Although it may be tempting in some relationships to "be the person my partner wants me to be," our experience has shown time and time again that misrepresenting our sexual needs and preferences will ultimately backfire. Before you can determine whether or not you're compatible with another person, you need to be honest about who you are and what feels right for you.

It is never too late for a woman to embrace herself and her sexuality. Cora made an appointment to see us because, at age fifty-six, she was seeking help in making intercourse more comfortable. Widowed for several years, Cora had recently begun a new relationship with a younger man—her first sexual relationship since her husband died. Now into menopause, Cora suddenly found that intercourse was not the same as she remembered. Becoming sufficiently lubricated was a problem, and as a result, intercourse was often uncomfortable, and sometimes actually painful.

When we asked Cora if she had shared this information with her boyfriend, she shook her head. "I'm just too embarrassed," she said. "I already feel self-conscious about my age, and I'm afraid if I talk to him about this, he'll leave me for someone younger."

While we recommended a course of lubrication for Cora, to be applied both before and during intercourse, we also encouraged her to discuss the subject with her partner and enlist his support. Rather than assume his reaction, we urged Cora to be authentic with her boyfriend and give him the opportunity to support her. Cora reluctantly agreed, and returned several weeks later with a glowing report.

"After meeting with you, I decided to be totally honest with my boyfriend. I told him that since I'm a bit older, I need a little extra lubrication, and that without it, sex was just not comfortable. He was surprised at first—he'd had no idea what I'd been going through—but he got right on board with the lubrication, and asked if he could be the one to apply it. Rather than it being a turn-off, I think it's been a turn-on for him to see me really enjoying sex for the first time. For me, I felt much freer just knowing I could be honest with him.

"Still, as powerful as the good feelings were," Cora confided, "I also felt very vulnerable, as though I'd been stripped of any protective covering. It felt frightening, but also somehow exhilarating. It took me fifty-six years, but I'm finally learning to be myself."

Without realizing it, Cora had described the paradox at the heart of sexual intimacy, which requires us to be vulnerable yet self-assured, honest about where we are yet open to changes. Indeed, being truly sexually connected to another person is not just a matter of technique, but the ability to be yourself, setting aside concerns about judgments, criticism, or comparisons.

You may be surprised to find out that being authentic is a turn-on for both of you. Regarding intercourse in particular, it is important for women to know that the vagina is host (or, in this case, "hostess") to the penis—a woman has the right to determine whether it will be invited in and how long it will stay.

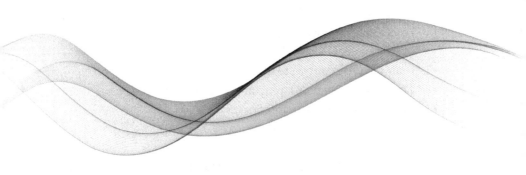

Chapter Seven

It's My Turn Now

Growing Through Menopause

What is Menopause?

Menopause is the name for the cessation of menstruation, which signals that a woman is no longer able to conceive. Though the process can begin in women as young as their late thirties, in most cases it takes place sometime in the mid-forties or fifties. For most women, menopause is a gradual process by which the ovaries diminish their production of estrogen, and the body slowly depletes its natural supply of estrogen. As a woman experiences this reduction in estrogen, she may notice a range of changes, both physical and emotional. (Generally speaking, a woman is considered to be postmenopausal beginning two years after her last period. However, for our purposes, we use the terms "menopausal" and "postmenopausal" interchangeably.)

While, of course, every woman's experience varies, the following are typical comments we hear:

- "Suddenly, I feel hot for no reason. Even my skin feels hot to the touch."
- "I can't sleep at night."

- "I feel really moody, like one long bout of PMS."
- "My vagina feels like it shriveled up!"
- "I can't have sex anymore! It hurts too much."
- "There's a constant dry, pinching sensation in my vagina."
- "I have to pee more often than before."
- "I feel anxious for no apparent reason."

While some symptoms such as hot flashes and sleep interruptions are well known and have even found their way into the popular lexicon, some of the most critical effects of menopause —loss of vaginal use, painful intercourse, urinary frequency and urgency, troubles with sex and sexuality—are rarely mentioned, let alone treated. Furthermore, most books on women's health tend to be geared toward the younger woman, and typically deal with menopause only in passing.

As a result, women may find themselves avoiding sex or suffering in silence, and/or forgoing regular pelvic exams when they become intolerable. (Our clinical experience suggests that difficulties with intercourse typically precede difficulties with pelvic exams.) It's not uncommon for healthcare professionals to simply hand women prescriptions for vaginal hormone replacements, assuring them that "everything will be fine," or to minimize women's concerns about menopause. In contrast, we like to remind women going through menopause that *knowledge is power* and that suffering need not be the inevitable solution.

We advocate for an approach that sees menopause as a natural stage of life, similar to other physiological milestones such as puberty or pregnancy. However, as with any major life transition, a lack of education may lead to feelings of isolation or confusion. Rather than attempt to ignore their symptoms and hope for the best, we encourage women to pay attention to the ways their bodies may be changing and, if necessary, seek appropriate treatment. Learning how to embrace and address these changes, rather than denying or ignoring them, can make all the difference in how a woman experiences this transition.

While in most cases menopause is a natural process, in other cases it may be brought on through surgical or chemical intervention. A woman who has undergone a complete hysterectomy and removal of her ovaries, for example, will experience the instant onset of menopause, irrespective of her age, as will women taking hormone-suppression medications for endometriosis, cysts, or uterine fibroids, and women treated for cancer. While the process of estrogen depletion during natural menopause is typically a gradual one, in cases when menopause is surgically or chemically induced, estrogen levels drop much more abruptly, which may result in aggravated and sometimes acute symptoms. While we hope this chapter will be helpful to any woman experiencing estrogen loss—no matter what the cause—we encourage women undergoing cancer treatment to consult Chapter Ten for additional information.

———

I Think I May Be Perimenopausal But I'm Not Sure. Aren't I Too Young?

Perimenopause is the timeframe of several years leading up to menopause during which a woman's menstrual cycle undergoes changes, ranging from less frequent periods to heavier or lighter flow. Natural perimenopause typically begins in a woman's early forties, though it can also begin in women in their late thirties. It is not unusual for a woman of thirty-six or thirty-seven who has started experiencing perimenopausal signs to ask us, "How can this be happening now? Aren't I too young?" While it may spark feelings of sadness or even loss, it is not at all unusual to begin to see a change in one's menstrual cycle as one approaches the end of one's thirties.

———

A Time of Changes

Upon entering menopause, it's not uncommon for a woman to notice a variety of shifts taking place in her body as well as in her mind. She may find, for example, that her vagina is less able to lubricate on its own, posing a challenge when it comes to intercourse or gynecological exams. She may feel a decrease in her general energy level, or find herself battling feelings of fatigue or depression. At other times, she may find that her moods are erratic and unpredictable, or perhaps she finds herself feeling anxious for reasons she can't articulate. As the estrogenic tissue surrounding the lower urethra thins out, it's also not unusual to experience an increase in the frequency or urgency of urination. Alongside any changes brought on by menopause, some women may also be dealing with other health concerns, from chronic back pain to arthritis to high cholesterol to some memory loss/word stumbling to weight gain, which may compound menopausal symptoms.

Women may also find that as their bodies change, so do their patterns of arousal. It may take longer to become aroused, or the orgasm may not be as strong. It is not unusual for women to discover that their orgasms simply aren't the same ones that they're used to; in less common cases, women may find they're unable to reach orgasm at all. Women may also begin to notice changes in the vagina itself. As estrogen levels decrease, there may be a diminishment in the size of the vaginal lips. This dip in estrogen also causes a woman's vagina to become less elastic, making her more prone to chafing, micro-tears, and infection. As a result, some women may experience some vaginal "spotting" after intercourse, which although typically benign (make sure to have it checked by your healthcare provider!), will naturally cause concern.

It has been our experience that various environmental factors may also contribute to feelings of vaginal discomfort at this time. For women who live in cold climates, the constant use of indoor heating systems can actually have a drying effect on the vagina, as can insufficient hydration caused by not drinking enough water. Certain medications, including those for allergies or anxiety/depression, may also compound the problem.

While these symptoms undoubtedly pose challenges, it's important to remember that they do not in and of themselves indicate any medical or physical pathology. Rather, they are simply the result of decreased estrogen, and can be seen as signs that the body is functioning properly, as it attempts to adjust to this new reality. The good news is that a sound restorative program should allow most menopausal and postmenopausal women to resume vaginal functions with little or no disruption.

Still, we don't deny that these shifts can be difficult, taking a toll on a woman's self-esteem. We encourage women to allow themselves to experience their feelings—of frustration, disappointment, or in some cases, grief.

At the same time, we try to remind women that change isn't always bad, and that "different" does not mean "bad," either. Sure, we might panic at first if we're not having the kinds of orgasms we're used to, but that doesn't mean the door can't be opened to new or alternative forms of intimate pleasure we hadn't previously explored.

Life does not end with menopause. On the contrary, with proper treatment and some effort, its effects can usually be managed, enabling women to continue leading full and active lives. In fact, women are increasingly coming to see menopause as an opportunity—a chance to reassess their choices and priorities, their health, and their relationships. As life expectancy continues to rise, we see more and more women taking advantage of the changes presented by menopause and middle age, with some using it as a time to take stock of who they are and who they want to be as they embark on the second half of their lives.

I've Lost All Interest in Sex. What Can I Do?

While menopause may hormonally diminish sexual interest, we are always delighted to hear menopausal patients who report "amazing sex" when they are in a new and exciting relationship, a phenomenon that emphasizes again and again that a woman's prime sexual organ resides between her ears . . . So what to do if you lose interest in sex? Explore the reason why—Boredom in the bedroom? Relationship problems? Too much on your plate to be able to shut off the thinking mind? We encourage women to take time to examine the underlying cause of sexual disinterest, enlisting the help of a therapist if necessary, so that they can begin to explore potential changes.

Am I Still a Woman?

As we get older, there's no question that things may look different in the mirror than they once did. We may have wrinkles that make us feel self-conscious, our breasts may sag a little, our backsides may not be as firm. And when it comes to such changes, we are often our own worst critics. If we're in a long term relationship like marriage, we may wonder if our partners still find us attractive. If we are new to the world of dating, we may question our desirability to a potential mate.

This is only natural, given that we live in a world that is saturated with images of young, toned female bodies, selling everything from beer to sunscreen. On television, online, in fashion magazines, and in the movies, we are continuously bombarded with the message that the twenty-something woman is the only feminine ideal. It is easy to compare ourselves and feel that we come up short. We may even fear that our partners will leave us for somebody younger. Knowing that we're no longer in our childbearing years, we may ask ourselves: "Am I still a woman?" The answer is, of course, a resounding yes.

We like to remind women that before anything else, *you have to learn to love yourself*. This is not achieved by ignoring reality, but by embracing it. It's a fact of life that our bodies at fifty-five will simply not look the same as they did at twenty-five. As women, we must remember that we are more than the sum total of our biology. With more years comes more experience, and with more experience often comes more wisdom. Certainly, we deserve, at any age, to be loved **and** appreciated for who we are, as we are.

What Can I Do About My Hot Flashes?

▸ Accept them as a natural component of menopause—knowing we can't always control nature.
▸ Pay attention to any anxiety they may trigger. We recommend taking a moment to relax your mind by taking a deep breath and reminding yourself that it will pass.
▸ Provide a cooler environment to ease the unpleasantness . . .

- Discuss with your healthcare provider whether a prescription for an SSRI (selective serotonin reuptake inhibitor) is a suitable option for you. SSRIs are a class of medications for anxiety and depression that have also been shown to help with "power surges."

Sex and the Menopausal Woman

When women ask us if it's possible to maintain an active, healthy sex life through menopause and beyond, we tell them, "Absolutely, as long as you're willing to make some modifications." In fact, not only is sexual activity possible, it's recommended!

We once received a call from a woman in her eighties who wanted to make an appointment to see us at our clinic. When she arrived, she explained that she had been happily married to the same man for over fifty years, and that they were currently enjoying a renaissance of sorts in their sex life. Her husband had recently received a prescription for Viagra, she explained, and she wanted to keep up with him. It was clear from the expression on her face and the light in her eyes that this was not a case of a woman subjugating herself to her partner's wishes but a situation in which two people were finding a renewed passion for one another later in life. And it wasn't only this woman's emotional state that was enlivened by her sex life; her vagina was in healthy condition too.

When a woman engages in intercourse through menopause and into postmenopause, her vagina will typically maintain a greater degree of elasticity, facilitating comfortable penetration as well as contributing to overall vaginal health. By way of contrast, a woman whose vagina is not sexually active during this time may find when she does decide to have intercourse, that penetration is painful, if not impossible. While we wouldn't go so far as to say it's a case of "use it or lose it," as one of our patients succinctly put it, there's no question that intercourse—as well as other forms of vaginal penetration—can help to maintain vaginal wellness as we get older.

It's important to remember that, as women, we're not the only ones facing changes as we approach middle age. Men are likely to find that their sexual capacities are not what they once were—whether it's a diminished libido, an inability to have or sustain an erection, or another health-related concern. They may find that they're struggling with a thinning hairline, a newfound paunch, or the prospect of retirement. While many men seem to take these changes in stride, others may find themselves questioning their identity and their manhood.

Confronted by a diminished self-image, or that of their partner, some older couples may find themselves opting out of sex altogether. This is a shame, since sexual intimacy can—and should—continue as long as we desire it. Communication between partners is vital at this stage. If at all possible, we advocate opening up a discussion with your partner about ways to maintain your sexual connection, so that you can embrace the next phase of your sexual journey together. We believe that the first step in this journey is acceptance. Simply acknowledging the fact that *our bodies have changed* will typically make couples more likely to take the necessary steps to ensure a mutually pleasurable experience.

In general, we tell older patients to be prepared for a little more planning when it comes to sex. The reason for this is twofold. In the case of men with erectile dysfunction, medications such as Viagra®, Cialis®, or Levitra® tend to take over an hour to kick in, which means some scheduling will come into play. As for the woman, lubrication should be embraced as part of *any* sexual activity, but is especially necessary when it comes to intercourse. We often remind women that it may not be enough to simply lubricate his penis before penetration or to apply a small amount of lubrication to the vaginal opening. Instead, we advise inserting lubrication directly into the vagina, using a vaginal applicator.

If your partner, for whatever reason, happens to object to the use of lubricant before or during sex, reassure him that it is not a commentary on his ability to arouse or please you, but that it is something that is necessary for your own vaginal health and comfort. You might also explain that the use of lubricant is more likely to ensure a satisfying experience for *both* of you. Remember: there is nothing wrong with advocating for your own needs, especially when it comes to your sexual health. If your partner remains dismissive or continues to outright object, it may be worth considering counseling to explore resolution and whether this is a person with whom you want to be intimate.

Of course, we can't talk about sex without talking about relationships. Today, it's not uncommon for women to find themselves newly entering the dating scene just as they're adjusting to menopausal changes, and it's perfectly natural to feel nervous about it, especially if the last time you did so was as a teenager! And yet, it's vital that we remember that we no longer have teenage bodies, meaning that some adjustments will most likely be necessary for comfortable intercourse.

If a woman has been paying attention to her body's changes, consulted with a health professional, and discussed any potential issues with her partner, her sexual encounter is more likely to be a positive one. If, on the other hand, she simply assumes that sex will work the same as it did when she was younger, she may be setting herself up for disappointment, as in the case of an email we received recently from a prospective patient named Kathy.

"I'm 50 years old and postmenopausal. I have been divorced for several years, and just started a new relationship. I was looking forward to enjoying sex with my new partner, but when he tried to penetrate me on two different occasions, he was unable to do so. Now he says he wants to call it quits! I don't know who to turn to for help. In all other areas, our relationship is going well. When it comes to sex, my desire is there, but my body doesn't seem to want to cooperate."

When Kathy came to our office for a consultation, she explained that she had already been to see her doctor, who promptly informed her that there was nothing he could do for her loss of vaginal elasticity, leaving her in a state of further despair. Acknowledging her disappointment, we explained that while decreased pliability and vaginal dryness are perfectly normal, there is no reason to live with pain, nor any reason to give up on a healthy sexual life. We told her, much to her apparent relief, that with supervised dilation therapy, vaginal elasticity is restorable.

Following our session, Kathy reported that while she wasn't sure that she wanted to continue her relationship with her current partner, at least she now felt confident that she knew how to respond to her body's changing needs. She said she felt relieved knowing that the next time she found herself wanting to be intimate with someone, she would know how to ensure it was a comfortable experience for her.

Unless a woman has remained consistently sexually active by way of sexual intercourse, we encourage menopausal women to use vaginal dilators if they wish to maintain vaginal elasticity for future sexual penetration, starting with a smaller size if necessary and gradually building up to one that corresponds to penis size, so that the vagina becomes accustomed to being stretched. We also recommend the use of a vaginal moisturizer, such as the over-the-counter Replens®, RepHresh®, Vagisil®, Luvena®, and Hyalo Gyn®. Lastly, we advise discussing with your healthcare professional the use of vaginal estrogen cream, the ultimate option for vaginal restoration, to be inserted inside the vagina and applied directly onto the vaginal lips and clitoris. Important: neither vaginal moisturizers nor prescription estrogen should be used during sexual activities, but rather inserted at bedtime and left to do their job while you sleep. Always remember to follow your healthcare provider's advice and the manufacturer's instructions.

What You Need to Know About Hormone Replacement Therapy

Oral hormone replacement therapy (in pill form) should be a matter of discussion between you and your healthcare provider because of the complex pros and cons of this intervention. In contrast, vaginal hormonal therapy, whether in the form of a tablet or cream, is a widely embraced intervention for the atrophic vaginitis of menopause and its associated urinary concerns[6], so be sure to see your clinician for evaluating your suitability and to discuss options.

6. Rahn et al. Vaginal estrogen for genitourinary syndrome of menopause: a systematic review. Obstet Gynecol. 2014 Dec;124(6):1147-56. Accessed January 05, 2015. http://www.ncbi.nlm.nih.gov/pubmed/25415166

We often see women who, after years of marriage, don't know how to advocate for their needs when beginning a new romantic relationship. After being out of the dating scene for decades, they oftentimes feel embarrassed or insecure about bringing up any sexual concerns with a prospective partner, or perhaps they simply can't find the words. Take the case of Eleanor, a woman who made an appointment with us on the suspicion that her new partner might have given her a sexually transmitted infection (STI). When Eleanor came to our office, we were shocked to learn that she had not insisted that her partner wear a condom. "I just didn't think it was that important," she told us. "He told me that, at his age, he just doesn't feel he needs to wear one anymore. At least, he said, we both knew there was no chance of me getting pregnant! And anyway, he's really such an honest, responsible guy. He was only with two other women before me . . ."

Eleanor sounded like a hormone-struck teenager rather than the educated professional woman in her early sixties that she was. When we asked her more about her background, it soon came out that her current partner represented her first foray into dating since her husband of many years had passed away several years earlier. "My husband and I were faithful to each other for forty years," she told us, "To be honest, I just don't have experience in things like this."

Still, as Eleanor spoke, we couldn't help thinking that something more complex was going on. All too frequently in our practice we see women who still feel that it's their job to "perform" sexually for their partner, regardless of what they're thinking or feeling inside. While Eleanor was reluctant to push her partner on the subject of condom use, another woman might be hesitant to let her partner know that a particular sexual position is uncomfortable for her, or to inform him that she needs additional lubrication before proceeding further. We encouraged Eleanor to establish a set of sexual boundaries for herself (for example, no sexual intercourse without a condom) and to maintain them. No woman, regardless of age, should allow herself to regress into silent suffering in an effort to "save" her partner's feelings. Rather than threatening to leave, as many women fear, it has been our experience that most men will respect their partner's decision to voice their own needs.

In Eleanor's case, she was lucky; it turned out she didn't have an STI. Yet, unfortunately, we've seen many sexually active older women who do. Often, with the possibility of pregnancy removed, women in middle age feel that they don't need to use condoms, mistakenly believing that sexually transmitted diseases "only affect the young." So let us take a moment to remind all the sexually active older women out there: **Until a new partner has been tested, condoms are still required!**

As was mentioned earlier, sex does not need to equal intercourse, and this is especially true as our bodies undergo physical and hormonal changes. If intercourse is proving to be too much of a challenge—or even if it isn't—we encourage couples to explore other forms of mutually pleasurable sexual stimulation off the Sexual Menu. This can include anything you and your partner agree on, from taking turns stimulating each other's genitals to sharing fantasies to giving each other massages to oral sex. It is important to remember that despite any changes occurring in the vagina, the clitoris is still your prime erogenous zone, and can be stimulated in countless ways, whether you're by yourself or with a partner. Many women report that they find themselves less inhibited as they get older, more willing to experiment with what excites them sexually. Whether or not you're currently in a partnered relationship, menopause is not the death of your sexual being. On the contrary, with some experimentation, you may find yourself having some of the best sexual experiences of your life.

Tips For a Healthy and Active Sex Life Through Menopause and Beyond:

▸ Lubricate for sexual intercourse.
▸ Moisturize the vagina to promote comfort and softness.
▸ Explore the option of vaginal estrogen for optimal restoration
▸ If his erection is affected, accept it as a fact of life and prepare accordingly.
▸ Embrace the sexual menu and its various options.
▸ Be prepared to adjust to new positions, as our bodies may move differently as we age.
▸ Practice safe sex and always use protection (condoms) until you are in an exclusive relationship and both partners have

been tested and cleared of sexually transmitted infections (STIs).

▸ Kegel exercises are an integral component of urogenital health and we encourage women of all ages to do them throughout their life cycles. Kegel exercises are especially valuable to menopausal women because of the natural weakening of the pelvic floor muscles and the diminishing muscle tone that is a normal part of aging. These changes may be contributing factors to organ prolapse, incontinence, and diminished orgasms, which is why Kegels are so important at this stage of a woman's life (see Chapter One for instructions).

I Feel Like I Just Woke Up...

Along with the physiological changes discussed above, many women find themselves going through other life changes as they hit menopause, and may discover they're at a crossroads. Perhaps they've recently been through a divorce or experienced the death of a spouse. Perhaps, with the kids grown or out of the house, they decide to embark on a new career path. In some cases, women may be considering reentering the work force after years spent raising a family. In other cases, women may suddenly find themselves caring for aging parents or facing a change in finances. As women continue to live longer, it is not unusual for us to find ourselves leading very different lifestyles than the ones we led when we were younger.

For some women, these changes can prompt difficult questions about purpose and identity. "What do I do now that my children don't need me anymore?" is a refrain heard from many women, as are questions like, "Who am I without my husband?" or "How do I make a living now that I'm on my own?"

Certainly, these changes in familial structure can be devastating for some women, plunging them into despair. Yet time and time again we have seen women come to us at middle age reporting a renewed sense of self, as they are no longer devoting all their energy to their husbands, kids, and homes. For many women, middle age brings opportunities that enable them, perhaps for the first time in their lives, to prioritize themselves, as illustrated in the case of Joy.

Joy, a woman in her early sixties, had spent the past thirty-five years of her life raising four children while enduring an unhappy and dysfunctional marriage. Joy had never worked outside the home and had devoted herself fully to her family, essentially raising the children herself, as her husband was emotionally distant and erratic. When Joy's youngest son left for college, she suddenly found herself alone in the house with her husband, questioning not only their relationship, but her purpose in life. Around this time, Joy's doctor informed her that she had high blood pressure and that if she did not start making changes, she would be placing herself at risk for heart disease.

Slowly, Joy began to reevaluate her life, beginning with prioritizing her health. She made modifications in her diet and began walking several miles every day—the first thing she had done just for herself in years. Feeling that she wanted to understand herself better, Joy began seeing a therapist, who helped her to realize how unhappy she was. After repeatedly disparaging her requests that they attend couple's counseling, Joy decided that she no longer wanted to remain in the marriage she'd been tolerating for so long. "As I got older, I realized I just didn't want to spend the rest of my life being with someone who wasn't there for me and didn't want to be. He was never a source of emotional support for me, even when the kids were little, but once they were gone, I had to ask myself how I wanted to live the rest of my life. To be honest, I feel like I just woke up."

Carol was happily married to her husband of thirty years and enjoying their empty nest together, when she began experiencing her first signs of menopause. "I realized I was getting older," she said, "and while I was very happy with my marriage, I'd been going to the same miserable office job for ten years and I couldn't help feeling I was wasting my life there." Carol was an avid cook and had always nurtured a dream of one day opening up her own small catering business. With the support of her husband, Carol gave notice at her job and enrolled in a local culinary school. "I feel like someone should pinch me," Carol says. "I'm finally living my dream. The only thing I can't help wondering is why I didn't do this sooner."

While some women fear the menopausal years as a time during which they come face to face with the fact that they are no longer defined by their husband and children, for other women, this may offer a sense of freedom, a chance to evaluate one's circumstances and goals. Joy and Carol are not the only women we know who found that, as they got older, they were more willing to take their own needs seriously.

I've Been Steadily Gaining Weight Ever Since I Started Menopause. Help!

Along with menopausal hormonal changes also come metabolic changes that translate into weight gain or difficulty losing weight. Furthermore, the common tendency to be less active as we get older may add to the problem. Quick tips include making changes to your diet or exercise program and ensuring you're getting proper medical care for managing associated illnesses that may be contributing factors.

Building Support

More than once, a woman has left our office saying, "All my girlfriends are going to hear about this." Whether she's referring to the fact that vaginal elasticity can be restored, the necessity of not suffering in silence, or the importance of inserting lubrication directly into the vagina before sexual activity, we find that more and more women are eager to share what they have learned about managing menopause. Unfortunately, it's still quite common to hear women tell us, "I thought I was the only woman going through this."

Because much of the medical establishment is still in the dark about how to address menopausal women's sexual concerns, it is vital that women share their experiences and knowledge with each other. This enables us not only to exchange tips and strategies, but also empowers our community of women facing similar struggles and victories.

As the years go by, many of us find that we value the support and camaraderie of other women more than ever. In fact, some of us may find that as we go through the hurdles of later adulthood, it is our girlfriends who remain a constant. Whether in the case of the death or divorce of a spouse, or simply the fact of having more time for oneself, old friendships are often rekindled during this time, while in other cases, hobbies or interests such as travel may pave the way for new ones. It is our belief that nurturing our connections with other women during this time can be yet another key factor in helping us successfully chart our way through this next phase of our lives.

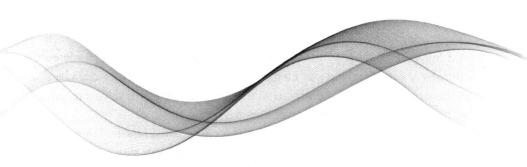

Chapter Eight

When Sex Hurts

Understanding Vaginismus, Dyspareunia,

Vulvodynia, and Vulvar Vestibulitis

In this chapter, we will explore the four most common conditions that make sexual intercourse painful, difficult, or outright impossible, and that affect untold numbers of women worldwide, many of whom suffer in silence, believing they are the only ones, unaware that their problem has a name, let alone a cure.

- **Vaginismus:** the inability to have, or great difficulty with, vaginal penetrations.
- **Dyspareunia:** painful intercourse.
- **Vulvodynia:** chronic pain in the vulva, with no identifiable cause.
- **Vulvar vestibulitis:** Vulvodynia localized in the vestibule.

Vaginismus, in particular, is a subject close to our hearts. For decades, we have specialized in this little-known disorder, treating women from all over the world at our New York practice. We wrote our previous book, Private Pain: It's About Life, Not Just Sex—now in its third edition—with the goal of bringing vaginismus into the open and raising global awareness about this "secret" problem. Our main hope then, as now, is to help sufferers feel seen and supported, and to let them know that there is a cure. Through updated editions of our book and our blog, we also aim to inspire other clinicians to learn more about this condition so that treatment will one day be readily available to to all women wherever they are.

Lastly, we have come to observe that the vagina often "speaks" our emotions, giving voice to the suppressed fear, anxiety, confusion, or sadness that countless women are unable to articulate directly, leading to emotional and physical breakdowns.

Vaginismus: A Vagina in Panic

Vaginismus (vag•i•nis•mus) is a vaginal penetration pain disorder characterized by the instantaneous, involuntary tightening of the pelvic floor muscles in anticipation of vaginal penetration of any kind. While some think that vaginismus is all about sex, that's not quite the case. The inability or great difficulty with vaginal intercourse is always present in vaginismus, but many women will also struggle with inserting a finger, wearing a tampon, undergoing a gynecological exam/vaginal ultrasound, or inserting a vaginal applicator for treating a vaginal infection. We call these the *Five Penetrations of Life*™. If you or a woman close to you has grappled with this condition, then you know the impact these restrictions can have.

Women with vaginismus often perceive their vaginas as "closed" or "blocked," and will typically describe any attempt at penetration as "hitting a brick wall." And indeed, because they are often also unable to insert their fingers to inspect their vaginas, many truly believe they have some kind of physical blockage.

In reality, there is definitely no "wall" inside the vagina. In fact, vaginismus is rarely caused by a structural limitation, but is, rather, triggered by feelings of fear and anxiety about the vagina or about penetration, which lead to an involuntary, reflexive clenching response. One could say that vaginismus is characterized by a breakdown of the relationship between a woman and her vagina. Unfortunately, vaginismus sufferers often report a kind of "vicious cycle of anxiety," in which worrying about their condition only makes it worse.

So it's no wonder that women will report feelings of inadequacy and isolation, along with the pervasive sense that their bodies have betrayed them. Nor is it surprising when our patients ask us, "Am I the only one suffering from this?" and "Will I be stuck with this forever?" Sadly, vaginismus remains a private condition, with most sufferers reluctant to talk about it.

When it comes to sexual intimacy, many women with vaginismus will have wonderfully satisfying sex lives without penetrative sex, while others will feel so anxious or unworthy that they avoid intimate relationships altogether. Still others will seek out—consciously or subconsciously—dead-end relationships that won't lead to sex of any kind. We have also encountered women who initiate break-ups—or behave in a way the encourages their partners to do so—as a result of their own shame that they cannot, as one of our patients put it, "do what a woman should do."

The feelings of confusion, loneliness, and frustration that result from living with vaginismus can lead to a sense of desperation. One of our patients, an accomplished athlete and baseball player, told us during her first treatment session that she sometimes hoped that squatting into the catcher's position "would cause something to rip down there so I could finally consummate my marriage."

There is no single "type" of woman who is diagnosed with vaginismus—and we have seen it all. At the time of this book's publication, we have treated over 1,200 women with this condition from all walks of life—Christian, Muslim, Jewish, Hindu, atheists, and more—from the U.S. and 29 other countries. Nor does vaginismus have anything to do with a woman's level of education or professional success—nearly 80 percent of our vaginismus patients are college-educated professionals, including gynecologists and other healthcare specialists. Sixty percent of them are married, while forty percent are single or in a relationship. Over half of our patients are between the ages of 26 and 35, approximately one quarter are under the age of 25, while the remainder are in their late thirties, forties, and fifties. The longest unconsummated marriage we have seen lasted 29 years; the couple ultimately had a child through assisted reproduction. Our youngest patient, age fourteen, came to our clinic because she wanted to learn how to use a tampon before she went away to summer camp. Our oldest patient, nearly sixty, had already lost two marriages due to her inability to have intercourse, and finally got tired of feeling like a prisoner in her own body.

Over the years, we've listened and held our patients' hands as they've told us . . .

- "It's like I'm not a real woman."
- "I feel trapped inside my body."
- "No one is as abnormal as me."
- "I've always thought of my vagina as dirty."
- "I don't know why my husband doesn't leave me."
- "I'll be the first case you cannot help."

You and your partner

There are lots of misconceptions about how men relate to women with vaginismus. Women who are dating are—understandably—reluctant to let prospective partners know about their condition on the assumption that "no man in the world would stick around for this," as one of our patients put it. Indeed, there remains an ongoing, widespread belief that men *must* have penetrative sex, and if that's not available on the Sexual Menu, there's no way they'll stay in the relationship.

And yet, the majority of men we have encountered in our practice care much more about their partner than they do about the missing penetrative sex. These partners remain supportive and committed, convinced they have found their soulmate. Valuing the deep friendship and bond that a loving relationship offers, they are willing to compromise sexually instead of leaving. Even in situations where the relationship ultimately ends, a lack of vaginal sex is not necessarily the primary reason.

While there's no question that sexual intimacy is a vital part of a relationship, whether it's between a man and woman or two women, there's also no question that sexual intimacy can be enjoyed through a wide variety of activities that are not at all affected by a woman's vaginismus. The bottom line is that vaginismus is by no means a death sentence for a relationship where genuine love and respect are present.

That said, women with vaginismus are not the only ones who suffer; if they are in relationships, their partners suffer as well, reporting their own sense of inadequacy, failure, and rejection. Some may wonder if the underlying problem is that "she does not love me enough." Female partners may wonder if they've "done something wrong," while male partners may have the sense that they are not quite "real men"—because if they were, then surely the problem would be solved by now. Inaccurate sexual information and a lack of understanding of the female body can worsen the crisis, sometimes leading to alienation, and the breakdown of the relationship. Here is how the boyfriend of one of our patients described his side of the experience:

> We were both virgins before visiting the Women's Therapy Center so neither of us had experience with penetrative sex. As a guy I wasn't used to being in a situation where I had sex with my partner every night so I didn't have an inherent expectation of intercourse. Before we found out about vaginismus, we were a very sexual couple and had enjoyed many other ways of stimulating each other. When we both believed it was the right time, we tried to lose our virginity to each other. As the millions of other couples around the world who have encountered vaginismus will have experienced, I wasn't able to slide myself inside my girlfriend, and felt discomfort and pain even though we were both aroused. We genuinely wanted to be doing what we were doing but our bodies were not cooperating or at least acting as expected. We both took our time, attempted it on different occasions and took advice from friends. We still had the same result. As I had not had any real previous sexual partners I was unable to know what we were doing wrong and doubted my ability to be a true man.

Primary and Secondary Vaginismus

There are two types of vaginismus: primary and secondary. Primary vaginismus is when a woman has never been able to have—or has always struggled with—vaginal penetrations. Secondary vaginismus is when a woman loses her ability to have vaginal penetrations at some point in her life. The causes for primary and secondary vaginismus are not the same, so let's examine each separately.

Contrary to a strongly-held misconception, sexual abuse is **not** at the root of primary vaginismus, though it can be a contributing factor in some cases. Instead, our statistics point to the following primary causes, in order of prevalence:

- Fear of pain upon penetration, in some cases resulting from stories shared by friends.
- Fear of the unknown: How will it feel inside? How will I react? What if I don't like the way it feels?

- Religious or cultural inhibitions and taboos.
- Fear of the vagina.
- Perceiving the vagina as fragile, susceptible to injury.
- Previous vaginal discomfort, whether from an infection, vaginal dryness, or an insensitive partner.
- Lack of education about sex and sexuality, including parental over-protectiveness.
- The inability to say no to unwanted sex.

In contrast to women with primary vaginismus, women with secondary vaginismus are able to remember a time when penetration was comfortable and effortless, until they underwent a particular lifecycle milestone or medical situation that threw their relationship with their body into havoc. These may include:

- Gynecological surgery,
- Menopause,
- Cancer treatment and radiation,
- Emotional or relationship crisis,
- Frequent painful urogenital infections,
- Sexually transmitted infections

Anxiety and vaginismus

It may not come as a surprise to learn that over 75 percent of our vaginismus patients have a legitimate anxiety disorder unrelated to their vaginismus, though not all have been diagnosed or been made aware of it. Such anxiety may affect the neck, back, intestines, head and jaw, emotions, relationships, and overall quality of life, as well as manifest itself as somatic ailments, and even an overactive gag reflex that can make swallowing pills difficult.

What does anxiety have to do with vaginismus? Well, the pelvic floor is connected to the stress response mechanism, meaning that the muscles react in times of stress by tightening and squeezing the vagina, urethra, and anus. Once such a stress association is established, it becomes a strong reaction of a **vagina in panic**. Keep in mind that the pelvic floor only becomes a "stress zone" when a woman has a negative association with sex, penetration, body image, and/or her relationship. To put it another way: the genitals are a component of the fight-or-flight response, our sympathetic nervous system that controls anxiety. For women with vaginismus, anxiety is channeled directly to their vaginas—though they may not even be consciously aware of it, and cannot control it.

Which brings us to the question . . . can anti-anxiety medications help? The answer depends on the level of a woman's anxiety: about half our patients do well without it, while the rest benefit from medication to curb the anxiety so that they can successfully proceed with the treatment. Of the latter group, some will continue taking medication even once cured, and may also begin psychotherapy to treat their generalized anxiety disorder. The medication route becomes even more essential if the woman has a history of panic attacks, depression, or OCD (obsessive compulsive disorder).

When presented with a recommendation for medication, patients may express concern that agreeing to it amounts to nothing less than "giving up," "taking the easy way out," or that it will somehow alter their personalities. As one of our patients told us, "Before I decided to go on anti-anxiety medications to fight vaginismus, questions circled in my head like vultures. What if I have debilitating side effects? What if I feel drugged all the time? Does this make me a less independent, less capable woman?"

Yet after successfully completing her treatment program, she reported a sense of satisfaction and empowerment she had never before experienced. "I was absolutely stunned to learn that my vagina was actually functional!" she told us. As for the decision to include medication in her treatment, she later wrote:

> "Meds are not a sign of personal failure; they allow you to finally do what you know you must. I learned that there was plenty left for me to do on my own. It was still extremely hard work, mentally and physically . . . Think of it this way: You're going to do battle with vaginismus and the medications are your armor. Wearing armor is no detriment to your fighting abilities. You are still going to need all the willpower and determination you can muster. It just means you're smart enough to recognize that when all your best instincts and intentions waver in the face of anxiety, your armor has your back, allowing a better, more capable version of yourself to emerge."

Myths and Facts

While the plain truth is that very few people have even heard of vaginismus, even among those who are familiar with the term, there remains a tremendous amount of confusion, lack of resources, unproven treatments, and frustration by patients and healthcare professionals alike. Consider the following examples:

- **MYTH:** *Keeping a dilator in your vagina overnight will solve vaginismus.* **FACT:** Stretching the vaginal walls does not help address the underlying anxiety associated with vaginismus, nor does it help the patient gradually acclimate to the sensation of penetration.
- **MYTH:** *Exercising your abdominal and lower-back muscles will solve vaginismus.* **FACT:** Vaginal penetration is unrelated to spinal/orthopedic health.
- **MYTH:** *You just need to relax.* **FACT:** If it were that simple, you'd probably already be cured! Treating this disorder requires addressing *both* the body and mind, including progressive, gradual, guided penetration training as well as anxiety management.
- **MYTH:** *Everything will be fine once you find the right guy.* **FACT:** Unfortunately, neither love nor sexual arousal can cure vaginismus. We have seen countless couples who are deeply in love, with plenty of sexual passion, but are still unable to have intercourse. Vaginismus is a condition that is about the woman herself, not about her partner.
- **MYTH:** *You can only be cured if you have a partner.* **FACT:** Single women can absolutely be cured from vaginismus with no less success than women in partnerships. This is because vaginismus is about a woman's relationship with her own body, not about her relationship with another person.
- **MYTH:** *'It's in your head, so just bear it . . . Get over it . . . Get used to it . . .'* **FACT:** Vaginismus may start in the head, but it translates into real physical pain.
- **MYTH:** *A hymenectomy will cure your vaginismus.* **FACT:** Opting for for a hymenectomy as a solution to vaginismus without first ascertaining the presence of an intact hymen is a widespread practice, which rarely results in a favorable outcome. Having

undergone a hymenectomy and still struggling with vaginismus is a major cause of patients' distrust and anger at the medical community.

Vaginismus and Pregnancy

The prospect of becoming pregnant and giving birth can present challenges for any woman, but it can be particularly challenging for women with vaginismus. The three most common questions we hear:

- Can I get pregnant if I have vaginismus?
- Will I be able to receive proper prenatal care if I have vaginismus?
- Can I give birth vaginally if I have vaginismus, and if so, does that mean I'm cured?

These are all excellent questions, so let's tackle them one at a time.

Can I get pregnant if I have vaginismus?

There remains a basic assumption that pregnancy can only occur as a result of vaginal intercourse, but that is actually not the case. The truth is that a woman *can* get pregnant if her male partner ejaculates by her vaginal lips during the week leading to ovulation, when the hormonal chemistry in her reproductive system is conducive to the sperm's survival. Additionally, we have met women with vaginismus who were able to conceive through assisted reproduction (infertility treatment) or by inserting their partner's semen into their vaginas with a small syringe. In other words, you can become pregnant without ever having vaginal intercourse, which means you are still a virgin. For this reason, we like to remind our patients who are not looking to become pregnant that **vaginismus is not a reliable method of contraception!**

Sadly, though, while many couples dealing with vaginismus are able to embrace the gift of pregnancy—and parenthood—we have spoken with others who report feeling like fakes, given that they did not conceive in the "normal" way.

Will I be able to receive proper prenatal care if I have vaginismus?

That depends on whether or not an internal gynecologic examination is possible. Given that most women with vaginismus are unable to tolerate a full gynecological exam, prenatal care will typically involve external physical exams only, and abdominal, rather than vaginal, ultrasounds. We advise doing your homework to find a knowledgeable and compassionate healthcare provider, and discussing with them how your vaginismus will affect your pregnancy and birth plan.

Can I give birth vaginally if I have vaginismus, and if so, does that mean I'm cured?

Typically, yes, you can give birth vaginally; and no, vaginal birth does not cure vaginismus. Your healthcare professional will usually opt to deliver the baby via Caesarean section (C-section) as a safe choice if vaginal examinations were not possible during pregnancy. For women who are able to tolerate gynecological exams, there is no reason they cannot give birth vaginally as easily and normally as a woman without vaginismus. As to curing vaginismus through vaginal childbirth, this is another fallacy that gives women false hope: vaginal childbirth is not a cure for vaginismus. Why? Because vaginismus is about entering the vagina, while childbirth is about exiting the vagina—two distinctly different body-mind functions.

Finding Treatment

It goes without saying that every woman suffering from vaginismus would like to overcome it and move on with her life. But the journey from here to there is rarely that straightforward. And for many, the long road towards healing is paved with ill-conceived "solutions" and frustrating attempts. Despite the proliferation of resources now available online, a woman's challenge in finding a cure is often compounded by the medical field's dismissive or ignorant attitude, with no standardized treatment, and a limited number of clinicians who understand the complex network of emotional and physical factors at play.

In this medical reality, misdiagnoses are common, most often with vaginismus mistaken for vulvodynia or vulvar vestibulitis. For so many of the women we have seen over the years, simply knowing that her inability to have penetration is not "all in her head" is immensely comforting. And the knowledge that she is not alone—that there are in fact thousands of women all over the world struggling with this very challenge—can sometimes be a vital step towards healing.

Some women with mild vaginismus—where the anxiety is not severe—are able to successfully self-treat using encouragement, relaxation, and vaginal dilators. For the rest, professional intervention is necessary for a complete and lasting cure. Such intervention will always require both physical and emotional management, based on an understanding of the body and mind as inseparable systems, each continuously influencing and being influenced by the other. For women who have finally grown tired of trying to pretend that nothing's wrong, or isolating themselves as a way to keep sexual relationships at bay, there is often tremendous relief in taking that first step by reaching out for professional help.

The emotional aspect of the treatment will teach the woman how to develop a sense of ownership over her vagina, including recognizing the associated anxiety and panic for what they are and resolving to never allow them to rule her life again. Easier said than done, right? Indeed, patience and expert guidance are needed to help build a harmonious relationship between the vagina and the anxious mind.

Of course, it's very common—and very understandable—for women suffering from vaginismus to feel apprehensive about treatment. Will it hurt? Will they stop if I ask them to? What if I'm the first failure? While powerful, and sometimes terrifying, this anticipatory anxiety is totally normal.

Many of our patients are pleasantly shocked to discover the ease with which they are suddenly able to experience vaginal penetrations. When it comes to intercourse, they will typically report later that "I didn't even feel it going in" or "I kept asking him if he was *really* inside me all the way." By the way: if a woman still doubts that he is fully inside her, we recommend that she feel for the penis by her vaginal opening; if she cannot feel any part of it, then it is completely inside.

The ease of the penis slipping into the now-cured vagina constitutes such a contrast to the memories of failed previous attempts, or of "suffering through it" in the past, that the relief and happiness our patients report is immeasurable. It's not unusual for them to say, "Is that what I was so worried about?" or "It wasn't as bad as I thought it would be!" One patient told us that following treatment, "I had so much more confidence. I walked taller. I felt like my marriage was 'real'" The simple truth is that no amount of reassurance can duplicate the empowerment of reclaiming the body, and finally feeling "normal."

Even women who overcome secondary vaginismus rejoice:

> The physical part was the easiest to overcome; I knew that I had been able to have sex before . . . with absolutely no pain, so I had to trust that my body could go back to what it used to be and it did. However, the emotional distress I gained, and all of the thoughts I was allowing my mind to have, have been hard to undo, and I still work very hard on not falling into my 'loop' . . . [Today] I am not scared (or if I am I try to be brave) and I confront life as opposed to hiding from it. I am enjoying sex again, and my relationship has gotten even better than it already was.

Of course, for women in partnerships, the benefits of treatment extend to their relationships as well. As couples are (finally!) able to explore and learn about intercourse together, they are afforded new opportunities for intimate closeness and communication. And indeed, couples who are able to overcome vaginismus as a team, often report that the challenge has strengthened their connection. Whenever possible, we like to include the partner—male or female—in a patient's road to recovery, and to listen to their feedback as well. Here is what a boyfriend had to say following treatment . . .

> I don't pretend to know for a second all the thought, fears, and internal turmoil that went on inside my girlfriend's head during the two years between finding out about vaginismus and getting to the Women's Therapy Center. I did, and still do, try as hard as I can to understand as much as possible . . . The treatment was only a couple of months ago and we're still exploring penetrative sex. We're not quite swinging from the chandeliers, but we're doing something that seemed unobtainable not so long ago. The emotional impact of vaginismus is still around but I hope it's lessening over time . . .
>
> If I had to say something to the partner of someone who's in the middle of vaginismus, I'd say that the seemingly impossible can be possible. It isn't just about the end result—it's about the journey. We never stopped being sexual towards each other and we're definitely a stronger couple because of vaginismus.

Vaginismus As A Gift

Is it possible that vaginismus has a silver lining? Impossible, you say? After all, vaginismus can destroy one's hopes and dreams, leaving women feeling humiliated and broken. Not to mention that most healthcare providers don't know what to do with it. So how can anything good come of it? In the early years of our practice, we might have agreed with this assessment. But having treated over twelve hundred women for this disorder, we have come to observe that there may indeed be a silver lining. While undoubtedly painful and demoralizing, living with vaginismus may nevertheless . . .

▸ Allow a couple time to develop their relationship.
▸ Protect a woman from being stuck with multiple children in a dysfunctional marriage/relationship.
▸ Afford a woman time to mature before embarking prematurely on marriage and/or motherhood.
▸ Offer an "out" in the case of an arranged marriage that doesn't work.
▸ Give a woman a reason to end an unhappy relationship instead of pretending everything's fine; she no longer needs to "settle."
▸ Delay childbearing only to discover later that there are conception problems or genetic risks, calling for alternative methods of becoming a parent.

Of course, we would never deny a woman her painful, despairing feelings when living with this dysfunction. Indeed, in the majority of situations, it is only possible to see the "gift" of vaginismus once a woman has been cured.

Understanding Dyspareunia

Dyspareunia (dys•pa•reu•nia) is just a hard-to-pronounce medical catch-all term that refers to difficult or painful intercourse. This difficulty can present itself at any point in the sexual encounter—at initial penetration, during thrusting, or following intercourse. Some women will feel pain at one of these points, while others will experience the entire process, from beginning to end, as painful. Like so many sexual conditions that affect women, dyspareunia is rarely discussed, poorly understood, and surrounded by shame. In reality, it is a multi-faceted phenomenon with a wide range of possible causes:

- **Medical causes.** These include vaginal infections, sexually transmitted infections (STIs), complications resulting from breast or gynecological cancer, various skin conditions, hormonal imbalances, intestinal or urinary tract problems, endometriosis, and more.
- **Physical causes.** These include changes in genital sensitivity as a result of menopause, size incompatibility, vaginal abrasions, scars, and/or nerve damage as well as complications from vaginal delivery.
- **Functional causes.** These include insufficient vaginal lubrication, genital irritations due to harsh cleansers and/or abrasive cleaning methods, poor hygiene, and friction irritation resulting from engaging in sports like cycling or horseback riding.
- **Psychophysical causes.** These can include everything from vaginismus to relationship difficulties to postpartum crisis.

Not surprisingly, dyspareunia can be a great source of anxiety in a woman's life—and a sensitive point of conflict in her relationship. Although intercourse is technically possible, the accompanying pain causes great distress; after all, who wants to suffer when it's supposed to be fun and enjoyable? For this reason, some women will do just about anything to avoid it, while others will suffer in silence, depriving themselves of the healthy intimacy that should be the cornerstone of their relationship.

The first step towards resolving the emotional and physical pain of dyspareunia is acknowledging to yourself that there is a problem. The second step is resolving to get help. Sadly, some women will resist treatment on the grounds that it's "too expensive" or "too embarrassing." Some women are doubtful there could possibly be a cure, while others hesitate to seek help out of fear that their partner will not support their process. Although the specific treatment plan will vary from woman to woman, the foundation of any course of healing will necessitate finding a competent clinician experienced with treating sexual pain disorders who will be able to conduct a thorough physical, emotional, and sexual evaluation to determine the most suitable intervention.

Understanding Vulvodynia

Vulvodynia (vul•vo•dyn•ia) is in incredibly prevalent disorder that manifests itself in countless women. Unlike other female sexual dysfunctions, it enjoys public exposure, medical awareness, large presence on the Internet, and insurance reimbursement, just like its subset cousin, vulvar vestibulitis (see below). Because the symptoms can be vague and inconsistent, and vary so much from woman to woman, it's not uncommon for women to doubt whether there is a problem at all and to put off seeking a remedy.

There are three types of vulvodynia conditions:

- Infectious vulvodynia, including candida, cyclic vulvitis, chronic vaginitis, as well as some herpes infections.
- Vulvar dermatoses, including lichen sclerosus, lichen planus, lichen simplex chronicus, erosive vaginitis, steroid rebound dermatitis.
- Dysesthetic vulvodynia, including vulvar vestibulitis. Also called idiopathic vulvodynia, which means vulvodynia without an apparent cause. This is the most common type of vulvodynia.

Infectious vulvodynia and vulvar dermatoses are diagnosed by a medical exam and/or laboratory tests, and typically respond well to prescription medication. Of note: in the case of lichen sclerosus, some women will need penetration intervention because of adhesions by the clitoris and the labia minora that limit or even prevent vaginal intercourse and pelvic examination with a speculum. We have had great success with such intervention, which allowed our patients to resume living normally without compromising their sexual practice and medical care.

In contrast, dysesthetic or idiopathic vulvodynia, the subject of this chapter, can be harder to diagnose and more difficult to treat. Because dysesthetic vulvodynia is such a complex condition, it requires an especially careful assessment by a knowledgeable, patient clinician who can help the patient find a resolution.

Depending on the individual, dysesthetic vulvodynia may present itself as one or more of the following:

- Burning, throbbing, itching, or stinging sensation in the vulva.
- Diffuse, generalized vulvar pain.
- The feeling that the vulva is being poked with needles.
- Urinary urgency and/or frequency.
- Associated stress-related conditions, such as irritable bowel syndrome (IBS), headaches, fibromyalgia, chronic fatigue syndrome, sleep difficulties, eating disorders, or temporomandibular joint dysfunction (problems of the jaw joint, often known as TMJ).

In our extensive work with dysesthetic vulvodynia, we have identified the following seven main causes for this distressing condition, each necessitating careful evaluation and personalized intervention:

- Vulvar dryness.
- Prolonged intake of antibiotics.
- Imbalance between the "good" and "bad" bacteria in the vulvar ecosystem.
- Excessive vulvar friction and irritation.
- Substance sensitivity or allergy.
- Inadequate vulvar hygiene.
- Hormonal changes.
- Emotional stress or trauma.

Unfortunately, not all vulvodynia sufferers can be helped by addressing the above causes, which lends support to recent understanding that points to physiological factors at the root of the disorder, including neural and immunologic conditions. As a result, a woman with dysesthetic vulvodynia may find herself caught in a seemingly endless cycle of pain, suffering, and depression. She may withdraw from relationships and sexual intimacy, avoid participating in regular life activities, and be angry at the medical field for being unable to diagnose or adequately address her symptoms. She may feel, as many of our patients once did, that she'll never be able to live a "normal life" again.

While these responses are perfectly understandable, we nevertheless encourage women caught in this cycle not to despair! Vulvodynia can often be resolved with the guidance of the right clinician—one who is willing to take the time to get to the root of the problem and create, together with the patient, a course of healing that takes into account both body and mind.

Understanding Vulvar Vestibulitis

Vulvar vestibulitis (vul•var ves•tib•u•li•tis), a subset of dysesthetic vulvodynia, is defined as a painful or irritating sensation in the vulvar vestibule. (The word "vestibule" simply means "entrance," and in this case refers to the area within the inner vaginal lips, where the entrance to the urethra and vagina are located.) Once again, the uncomfortable sensation that characterizes this condition will vary, and may manifest itself as one or more of the following:

- The feeling of being cut at the bottom of the vaginal opening (sometimes called the "6 o'clock spot").
- Tenderness, swelling, or rawness.
- Burning, stinging, itching, dry, or "hot" feeling.
- Pain upon contact, including underwear and tight-fitting clothing.
- Urinary frequency.
- Severe pain upon attempted vaginal penetration.

As with any genital dysfunction, these symptoms will disrupt a woman's quality of life, leading her to distance herself from potential intimacy, and for some, resulting in a full-blown emotional crisis. Although many hypotheses have been suggested as to the cause of this condition, the medical community has yet to arrive at a consensus, resulting in a range of interventions, including everything from topical medications and anti-depressants to cognitive-behavioral and biofeedback therapy, laser surgery, even Botox injections.

Vulvar vestibulitis has an array of potential causes that are similar to dysesthetic vulvodynia, including:

- Insufficient hydration.
- Prolonged intake of antibiotics.
- Insufficient lubrication.
- Emotional stress.
- Allergy or substance sensitivity.
- Structural, chemical, hormonal, or environmental causes.

As with dysesthetic vulvodynia, there is ongoing research suggesting that physiological factors may also play a role in the disorder. Either way, the good news is that once a woman's particular cause is identified and her customized treatment plan implemented, she should begin to feel improvement. As always, we advocate a body-mind approach to healing, given that both a woman's body and mind are affected. Of course, every woman will have her own individual journey of prognosis and recovery, but ultimately, there is no reason she cannot return to feeling like herself again and resuming sexual intimacy.

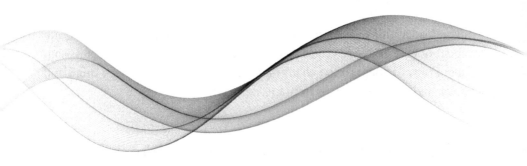

Chapter Nine

Healing the Sexual Scars of Cancer

While many of the topics addressed in this book will apply to most women at some point in their lives, cancer is something that none of us hopes to ever encounter. And yet, increasingly, it is not unusual to find ourselves touched by cancer in some way, whether we're providing support to a parent, spouse, child, sibling, or close friend as they undergo treatment and its aftermath, or we're facing our own diagnoses, attempting to find our way through a labyrinth of treatment options and emotions, while wondering if our lives will ever be the same again.

Facing a cancer diagnosis is never easy, even when the prognosis for recovery is good. Women dealing with cancers that affect their sexual organs, whether directly or indirectly, face a particular set of challenges. This group of cancers is comprised of breast, bladder, and gynecologic cancers, including cervical, endometrial, uterine sarcoma, fallopian tube, ovarian, vaginal, vulvar, and Gestational trophoblastic disease (GTD). For the sake of clarity, we will collectively refer to them as "female cancers."

Being diagnosed with a female cancer forces a woman to confront not only the illness itself, but also the question of who she is now as a woman. Even in cases of early detection and successful treatment, women will often find themselves feeling that their identities have been compromised, as they struggle to adjust to their post-cancer bodies and spirits.

We have written this chapter specifically with the female cancer patient in mind, aiming to address not only the cancer, but how a woman can go on to lead as full a life as possible once it's been treated. This chapter is not about how to eradicate cancer—we'll leave that to your medical team—but about how to adapt to the changes it brings about in a woman's mind and body, and emerge stronger from the experience.

What Your Healthcare Provider May Not Tell You

Often, female cancer patients are not informed about what to expect in terms of how their bodies will change following treatment, particularly when it comes to sexual function. As one of our patients put it, "Having cancer was hard enough. Now, after all that, to find out my vagina isn't working the way it used to—I just feel so cheated and so angry." Indeed, while modern healthcare has made great strides in treating the disease, there are still gaps in addressing patients' post-treatment sexual and emotional needs.

How a woman's sexual health will be impacted by cancer and/or cancer treatment will be determined by a range of factors, including what type of cancer she has and how advanced it is; her family history and genetics; her general state of physical and emotional health pre-diagnosis; her lifestyle habits; and what kind of support system she has in place. Some cancers will target the reproductive system/genitals directly, while others will exert indirect effects. Either way, we advocate for an approach that takes into account the patient as a whole, not merely her specific body parts.

When it comes to treating cancers that directly affect a woman's sexual organs—such as uterine, cervical, vulvar, vaginal, bladder, or ovarian—what can women expect?

- Following **surgery**, the vagina may be shorter, less elastic, more tender, and may develop internal scarring or adhesions.
- **Chemotherapy** typically throws a woman into abrupt menopause, bringing about the urethral, vaginal, and sexual changes, including vaginal dryness and decreased elasticity; thinning of vaginal tissue, which can lead to a tendency to tear and ulcerate easily; increased urinary frequency; dyspareunia (painful intercourse); and overall urogenital atrophy.
- Both, surgery to remove the ovaries and pelvic **radiation** will induce menopause as noted above. Additionally, the irradiated

skin will become thin and/or brittle and dry, similar to a burn injury; it may easily tear, chafe, or bleed upon contact, especially during or following sexual penetration or the use of vaginal dilators. Radiation may also result in the formation of scars or adhesions that will restrict some or all of the vaginal canal, the most common being the "hourglass adhesion," which creates midway closure of the vagina. Radiation may also irritate the bladder, leading to discomfort and increased urinary urgency, and form scars or adhesions around the intestines, leading to intestinal problems. Scarring/adhesions in and around the vagina may also cause pain during orgasm.

Why Me? The Emotional Challenges of Cancer

Beth was a busy young mother of three little girls who was simultaneously studying for her graduate degree in psychology when she was diagnosed with ovarian cancer. Three months after completing her radiation treatments, she came to see us for vaginal restoration therapy.

Vaginal dilation treatments proved extremely effective for Beth, especially because she made an appointment while her vagina was still pliable and in functional condition. As long as she remembered to stretch her vagina before intercourse using the dilation method, she found that her sexual life with her husband continued uninterrupted. Beth was grateful that she had sought treatment and was able to continue to be close with her husband, exploring their intimate zone in new ways that became no less satisfying than prior to cancer. Maintaining this connection, Beth explained, provided a touchstone for both of them, given all they had been through in the past year. Still, despite her successful physical recovery, Beth could not shake the feeling that she'd been victimized by cancer. Even as her body was making the necessary adjustments to life posttreatment, Beth remained haunted by the question of how her family would have coped without her.

"I lie awake at night and think, 'Who would have taken care of my daughters?'" she told us one day. "Now that I am here, I feel like I have to give them every second of every day because I don't want to miss out on anything. But the truth is, I think I'm suffocating them, and I don't feel very happy myself."

By then, Beth had passed the two-year mark of being cancer-free, but she still had yet to *free herself* from the frantic sense that she must live every day as her last.

Other women may be facing a very different set of concerns. Recently married and in her early thirties, Elisa and her new husband had always dreamed of having a big family. When Elisa was diagnosed with leukemia, she and her husband were initially devastated, only to find that within a year, her radiation and chemo treatments had been successful and she was fine.

"We thought it was going to be a time to celebrate," Elisa said when she came for an appointment. "But then, suddenly, I realized that my body was going through menopause and within a short time, we found ourselves sitting in yet another doctor's office, this time being told we'd never be able to have children. The elation I felt at having survived cancer has now been totally eclipsed by my devastation over the fact that I'll never be able to conceive."

Indeed, the inability to conceive and/or have biological children can be a terrible blow. However, if being a parent is something that's important to you, it's vital to know that you have options. These include egg retrieval prior to surgery/treatment, fertilization using a donor egg, or adoption. The most important thing to remember is that biology is not necessarily destiny, and that with today's fertility advances, there are numerous ways to become a parent.

There are countless emotions that a woman may experience as she navigates her way through cancer: anger, resentment, fear, and grief, to name just a few. We've had more than a few women ask us, "Why me?" Unlike other physiological changes we may have undergone throughout our lives, such as pregnancy or menopause, there is often a sense with cancer that *our bodies have betrayed us*. We may feel angry at God or at ourselves, trying to figure out what we did "wrong." Forced suddenly to confront questions of life and death, we may find that we feel overwhelmed, anxious, or depressed. If a woman has already been struggling with anxiety or depression, she is likely to be additionally challenged.

Cancer affects each of us differently. Depending on age and life circumstances, we may be concerned about how cancer will impact our relationships with our partners—or with prospective partners if we're single. If we have children, we may wonder whether and how to break the news to them, or worry about being a burden. If we don't have children, we may be facing the reality that we will not be able to become biological parents—an especially difficult challenge for women who receive a cancer diagnosis during their reproductive years. If we are caring for aging parents, we will likely feel anxious about who will take care of them in our absence.

With medical urgency as their ultimate priority, it is rare that healthcare providers address their patients' emotional needs at the time of diagnosis, leaving them unprepared for the challenges ahead. To bridge this void in patient education and support, we encourage women to seek out a qualified therapist or counselor to help guide them through the emotional upheavals that are so commonly experienced at this time. Our clinical experience with cancer patients has shown us time and time again that it is not enough merely to address a woman's physical needs, but her psychological needs as well.

Some of our patients have also found comfort and community in attending cancer support groups, whether in person or online, which can provide a vital opportunity for sharing experiences with those facing similar struggles. Other women we know have used their diagnosis as a catalyst to reconsider their lifestyle choices—everything from health and relationships to faith, career, hobbies, and level of physical activity. Ideally, cancer management should be viewed as a process—a process that needs to be supported from both a medical as well as mental health perspective—from the time of diagnosis, through treatment, and beyond, as we begin to gradually rebuild our lives with cautious optimism.

An integral part of this process is coming to grips with the fact that cancer has altered our lives. There tends to be little space in our culture for such feelings, which is why it is so important that we create safe spaces where they're permitted. We encourage women to allow themselves a process of grief, acknowledging their pain and despair. We counsel women to remember that *experiencing feelings of sadness or loss does not make you a victim.*

Sex and Cancer

When Paula arrived for her initial visit, she promptly informed us that she was at her wit's end. A professional woman in her mid-forties, she had recently completed a successful round of radiation treatment for uterine cancer. She was six months cancer-free, and her healthcare provider assured her that she was in the clear.

"The problem," Paula told us, "is that I can't have sex."

Paula had a boyfriend of several years, and though he had been a steady source of support during her treatment, spending countless hours at her bedside while she was nauseated or exhausted, she felt that he was beginning to lose patience.

"John and I didn't have sex for nearly a whole year," she said. "I always felt too sick, and he really seemed to understand. But now time has passed and he wants our lives to get back to normal. I keep telling him I want that too, but it just doesn't seem possible. I'm starting to worry that if we can't have sex, he'll leave me—and I can't say I really blame him."

When we asked Paula if her healthcare provider had prepared her for the fact that the volume (i.e., length and depth) of her vagina would be affected by radiation, she told us that at her final treatment, her radiologist simply gave her a brown paper bag containing a vaginal dilator and told her to use it.

"There were no instructions or explanations," she told us. "I guess he just assumed I'd figure it out on my own. But I had never seen a dilator in my life, let alone used one, and it looked terrifying! I put the brown paper bag in my closet and never touched it again."

The first thing we told Paula was that she is not alone. Following surgery, radiation, and/or chemotherapy, it's not uncommon for a woman to find that sexual intercourse is difficult, if not impossible, as her vagina is simply no longer able to house the penis, let alone its thrusting motion. She may also feel anxious about whether intercourse will be painful, and/or cause further damage to her already sensitive vaginal tissue. A woman may encounter this reality in the context of a sexual experience, such as intercourse or penetration with a dildo, or she may discover it on a visit to her gynecologist, even if she'd been able to have posttreatment pelvic exams in the past.

This difficulty with penetration will understandably leave her feeling despairing and frustrated—or, as Paula put it, "like half a woman." In Paula's case, her feelings of low self-esteem were compounded by the fact that she had put on weight as a result of trying to medicate her low mood with food, which in turn added to her anxiety that her boyfriend would leave her.

The good news, we told Paula, is that vaginal elasticity and function are usually restorable through a guided program of dilation therapy and vaginal lubrication. We also recommended that she meet with an Oncology Social Worker (a psychotherapist who specializes in cancer) to help her sort through her body and relationship concerns. Happily, this combination of therapies worked for Paula, and within several months of her initial consultation, she was reporting increased self-esteem and improved communication with her boyfriend, with whom she was now able to have comfortable intercourse, much to their mutual delight. Still, these positive changes were not without effort. In order to continue on this path, Paula had to commit to maintaining a regular program of dilation therapy at home, and remembering to always generously lubricate in advance of any sexual activity.

In other cases, as a result of resistant adhesions, vaginal restoration through pelvic floor physical therapy and/or dilation may simply not be possible. If medically suitable, some women with adhesions will opt for corrective surgery to remove them, commonly referred to as a "clean-up," while others will require more involved reconstructive surgery. Although there are women who have successfully undergone such procedures and found them helpful, there are others who have decided that such elective surgery is not for them. It's important to remember that there is no right or wrong when it comes to making this personal decision, which we encourage each woman to make for herself.

In these situations, and in others in which intercourse is physically impossible for other reasons, couples are encouraged to find new ways to maintain their sexual intimacy. This is the time to consider the Sexual Menu and begin exploring alternate forms of sexual pleasure to enjoy with one's partner. As we always like to remind our patients: **Just because you can't have intercourse, doesn't mean you can't have a mutually satisfying sex life.** Many couples find they are able to enjoy other kinds of sex, including modified intercourse, in which the penis penetrates the vagina only partially, or thrusts close to the vaginal opening while the woman squeezes her thighs around it. Remember: a woman's erogenous zone is her clitoris (located north of the vagina!), which means that there's no reason that any changes in her vagina should affect her capacity for sexual pleasure, even if her orgasms have become less intense.

A woman's ability to have open communication with her partner at this time can be a major determinant in whether she is able to embrace her post-treatment sexual identity. Women who are able to talk with their partners about their bodies' changes and altered physique will, naturally, be better prepared to make the necessary adjustments to their sex lives. As always, we maintain that knowledge is power. The more informed we are about our bodies' changes, the better we'll be able to explain them to our partners and enlist their help in working through the changes together.

While making adjustments to our sex lives is not always easy, let's remember that the human body is in fact quite resilient, with the most wonderful abilities to restore itself when given the proper help. For most women, this is a process that will require time, patience, and practice. The most important thing is not to be afraid of your body. As long as a woman has clearance from her healthcare provider, we urge her not to hesitate to challenge herself. In most cases, our bodies are a lot stronger than we think.

When Your Partner Has Cancer

Supporting a spouse or partner with cancer presents myriad challenges to us as individuals as well as to our relationships. Beyond the day-to-day logistics of managing the household and family, there is also attending doctors' appointments, dealing with paperwork, and spending nights at the hospital, all likely to trigger countless emotions, from fears of abandonment to anxiety about the future. Depending on the type of cancer your partner has, and his or her chosen course of treatment, you may also find yourself negotiating the new realities of your sexual relationship.

Men who undergo treatment for cancers in the pelvic or lower abdomen— colorectal, bladder, or prostate—will often develop urinary incontinence, Erectile Dysfunction (also known as ED, the inability to attain or sustain an erection), and the effect of burned, irradiated skin, which may make intercourse impossible, even if the erection is unaffected.

As a partner, the first thing you need to appreciate is how devastating this is for him because of the paramount importance of penile function to a man's identity, a breakdown that may lead to profound anxiety and/or depression, making it difficult to maintain intimacy. Men will typically sum up their experience by saying, "Who am I without my penis?" A woman's attempt to convince her partner that the loss of intercourse is okay with her may be futile, given that the male sexual template is so different from hers. Because of this difference, it is worth noting here that lesbian couples are typically better prepared to handle the sexual changes brought on by cancer treatment.

Men may need to be coaxed to discuss their sexual crisis with their healthcare provider and map out an appropriate treatment plan, which may include ED drug therapy (i.e., medications such as Viagra®, Cialis®, Levitra®, Staxyn®, or Stendra®), sexual counseling with a male clinician, male support groups, etc. When needed, we urge couples to find an experienced psychotherapist who can help them negotiate the heightened emotions that accompany such profound personal changes.

Vaginal Wellness: Tips and Suggestions

As we've mentioned throughout this chapter, a program of regular, supervised vaginal dilation therapy is indispensable for maintaining vaginal wellness both during and following female cancer treatments. It's important, however, for women to know that there is a time factor when it comes to beginning a rehabilitative program, as the vagina will tend to lose flexibility within two to three months of undergoing treatment. For this reason, we encourage women to start a restorative/therapeutic program as early as they are permitted to do so by their healthcare provider. While dilation therapy can be done at home (as long as one is not afraid to do it!), we recommend first consulting with your medical team or with a pelvic floor physical therapist who specializes in treating cancer patients for initial guided instructions, including proper lubrication.

In addition to dilation therapy, the following are useful suggestions for maintaining genital and sexual health during cancer treatment and posttreatment. However, these suggestions are not a substitute for medical advice; consult with your healthcare provider before undertaking any of them:

- Internal vaginal lubrication to counter dryness during penetration. We recommend using an applicator to insert the lubrication into the vagina prior to intercourse or dilator use to ensure lubrication will last throughout the activity.
- To alleviate genital dryness or stickiness of the genital lips, apply Aquaphor® Healing Ointment 1-3 times daily. It can also be used on the vaginal opening if the area feels uncomfortably tight, and around the anus in cases where radiation has irritated the area.
- The drop in estrogen levels, combined with radiation treatment, may make your urethra more sensitive to chafing during vaginal penetration by penis or dilator, and may also bring about urinary urgency. You may want to strengthen it by drinking 1-3 cups of Stinging Nettle tea daily, and taking live probiotics in capsule form on a daily basis. Probiotics are also great resistance fighters against yeast and urinary tract infections, and a wonderful support to the digestive system.
- In cases where your healthcare provider has advised against vaginal estrogen replacement, try nourishing your vagina at bedtime with an estrogen-free, long-lasting vaginal moisturizer such as Replens®, RepHresh®, Vagisil®, Luvena®, or Hyalo Gyn®. *Remember: These products are not a substitute for using a lubricant during intercourse!*
- If you are undergoing radiation, especially internal radiation, obtain clearance from your medical team for the use of daily vaginal lubrication/moisturizer options such as K-Y® jelly or Replens®, RepHresh®, Vagisil®, Luvena®, or Hyalo Gyn® to soothe the vagina and help to maintain its elasticity as much as possible. You may also want to discuss the use of Aquaphor® Healing Ointment on the external genitals/anus, and taking the above-mentioned nettle tea and probiotics.
- If you're in a relationship, discuss and explore the changes your body is going through with your partner so that you can adjust your sexual activity accordingly. This may include lubrication, pre-penetration dilation, modified sexual positions, different sexual activities, adding sexual toys, etc.

The Search For the Silver Lining

Kelly was a woman in her late thirties who came to see us for vaginal restoration, having recently finished a series of chemotherapy treatments for aggressive uterine cancer. As we went through her personal and medical history, Kelly shared that she had been married for ten years to a wonderful man.

"My husband and I have always had a strong marriage," she told us. "But ever since my diagnosis, I feel like our relationship has grown and deepened in ways I never could have anticipated. Even though it was definitely the hardest thing either of us has ever gone through, I think we both feel a renewed appreciation for each other. Now that the cancer is behind us, I know I'll never take our time together for granted."

Kelly is just one of dozens of women we've seen over the years who was able to discover what we call "cancer's silver lining." While the ability to see the hidden gifts in a given situation is helpful in dealing with life's ups and downs in general, it is particularly valuable when confronting cancer. There's no question that cancer will drain us physically, emotionally, and sexually. As we've discussed, we implore women to take the time to create a safe space where they can allow themselves to feel their painful feelings—whether by themselves, or with a partner, therapist, or trusted friend. At the same time, our clinical—as well as our own personal—experience has shown over and over that cancer is all about how you look at it.

Indeed, the ability to find something positive in one's diagnosis, no matter how bad it may seem, is often a key factor not only in surviving cancer, but in embracing life posttreatment. Cancer often serves as a wake-up call for women, prompting them to reevaluate their relationships with their partners, their families, and themselves. Over the years, we've seen women who chose to see cancer as an opportunity to begin to make new choices, whether it's getting out of a dysfunctional relationship, taking better care of their health, or reconnecting with important people from their past. Or, as in Kelly's case, to simply embrace more closely what she already has.

Sometimes cancer may serve as a catalyst for us to push ourselves in new ways, both big and small.

"When I first found out, I was so angry," explained Rona, a woman who was diagnosed with uterine cancer in her mid-fifties. "I couldn't understand how this could happen to me. But as the months passed, I had to ask myself:

Was I just going to continue being angry, or was I going to find some way to work through it?"

Rona regularly took a cab to and from her radiation appointments in New York City. One day, she decided that instead of taking a cab home as she usually did, she would walk downtown to meet her son for lunch. This was no simple thing, as the walk from the hospital to her son's office was nearly a hundred blocks.

"I'd never walked that far in my life," Rona told us. "But I was determined to do it. I had to prove to myself that my body still worked."

Not only did Rona's new approach help to clear her mind (and save her cab fare!), it also proved to her that her body was still strong and capable. In the meantime, her weekly lunches with her son became a treasured time for both of them, an oasis amidst the cancer madness.

"I needed to find a way to feel whole again," Rona said, "and this was, literally, a first step."

Epilogue

s women, our sexuality is a complex web that includes not just our hormones and genetics, but also the messages we received from our parents, our teachers, the media, and the whispered information gleaned from older friends. The attitudes we were exposed to growing up play a key role in determining how we understand and navigate the sexual dimension of our lives. Do we see sex as an avenue to connect with someone we love, or do we see it as part of a series of obligations we undertake as partners, wives and mothers? Are we able to explore our sexual impulses and desires on our own terms, or do we believe that sexuality only has a place within the confines of marriage?

The starting point for our understanding of women's sexuality is its being a natural, physiological function. Our sexual desires and impulses comprise one of the most basic and essential parts of who we are as individuals. At the same time, our emotional needs cannot be separated from our physical response. When we feel that our needs as an individual are being taken into consideration--when we feel cared for and listened to—we are able to feel safe enough to let go, and let pleasure in. When we feel exhausted, burnt out, or taken for granted, our bodies will speak for us, making sex either impossible or indeed just another "chore" to get through.

Let us remember that a sexual relationship with another person has the potential to yield more than children. It can be a source of comfort, connection, and—dare we say it—pleasure.

Thus, we affirm a woman's right to making her own sexual choices and ask you to help us carry the message that sexuality is a gift—something to be enjoyed and celebrated—at all stages of a woman's life, regardless of her age, religion, sexual orientation, or relationship status.

Resources

Note to our readers: with Internet search providing endless in-depth resources, we limited the following to a short list of key entries.

Vibrators

1. Vibrators come in different sizes, shapes, and materials; some will be for use inside the vagina while others are for clitoral and vulvar stimulation only.
2. Generally speaking, hard materials (plastic) will transfer vibration more efficiently (strong), while soft materials (rubber, silicone) are gentler. Choose the one/s that feels right for you.
3. You may want to use a condom on vibrators made of silicone or rubber because they are porous in texture, which may not allow for adequate washing after use.
4. When using a vibrator on the clitoris, always remember to use lubrication!
5. Where to buy vibrators? At sex shops, or online (do an Internet search, and look for vendors with discreet shipping labels).

Vaginal Applicator

1. An applicator comes with vaginal preparation. It can be reusable, or disposable (for one time use only).
2. For an in-depth description of how to use and clean an applicator, read our Blog post titled *Vaginal Applicator* at www.womentc.com/blog
3. Should you need to purchase additional applicators: you can either buy a vaginal preparation, i.e. for yeast infection or for lubrication, and use the applicator it comes with, or buy one on the Internet by searching for either a reusable or a disposable vaginal applicator.

Ovulation, Conception, Pregnancy

- American Pregnancy Organization
- BabyCenter.com
- Pregnancy: The Ultimate Month-by-Month Pregnancy Guide, by Dr. Anne Dunn
- The Pregnant Body Book, by DK Publishing

Conception & Pregnancy Apps

- DigitalOrientation.com
- My Days—Period & Ovulation
- My Cycles Period and Ovulation
- BabyCenter My pregnancy Today

Menopause

- The North American Menopause Society

Contraception, Sexually Transmitted infections, Abortion

- Planned Parenthood
- Womenshealth.gov

Cancer

- Foundation for Women's Cancer
- National Cancer Institute
- American Cancer Society
- BreastCancer.Org
- LiveStrong.Org

Index

About the Authors

Ditza Katz, PT, PhD, is the founder of Women's Therapy Center, a practice specializing in urogynecologic rehabilitation, treatment of female sexual dysfunction, breast & female cancer rehabilitation, and management of somatic disorders.

Dr. Katz holds an undergraduate degree in Physical Therapy, a Master's degree in Pastoral Psychology & Counseling, a doctorate in Clinical Sexology, and clinical training in manual therapy and urogynecology.

Dr. Katz is a Diplomate with the American Board of Sexology, Clinical Assistant Professor at the American Academy of Clinical Sexology located in Orlando, Florida, and is the only physical therapist in the USA who is a clinical sexologist.

Ross Lynn Tabisel, LCSW, PhD, is Co-Director of the Women's Therapy Center and a Diplomate with the American Board of Sexology.

She holds a Master's degree in Social Work from Adelphi University, a Post-Graduate Certificate in Psychotherapy and Psychoanalysis from the Institute for the Study of Psychotherapy in New York, a doctorate in Clinical Sexology, and Certificate Training in the area of Sexual Abuse.

Dr. Tabisel is the first Social Worker to be accepted as a member of the American Urogynecologic Society and of the American College of Obstetrics and Gynecology on the merit of her expertise. She is a Board Certified Diplomate in Clinical Social Work, and Clinical Assistant Professor with the American Academy of Clinical Sexology located in Orlando, Florida.

Together, **Dr. Katz** and **Dr. Tabisel** pioneered the **DiRoss Methodology**^{SM}, a successful intervention for vaginismus and dyspareunia, for which they have become known worldwide. Because of their expertise, they have been invited lecturers, nationally and internationally, educating healthcare professionals about their unique team approach to female sexual dysfunction. Media appearances include Discovery/ TLC TV and Oprah Channel, NBC's Nightly News, SexTV (Canada), Glamour, Lifetime Online, Newsday, and more.

Visit their website (www.womentc.com) for in-depth information concerning female genital and sexual health, and for professional biography, speaking engagements, media appearances, publications, and training.

Made in the USA
Middletown, DE
31 March 2021